FOOD IS YOUR BEST MEDICINE!

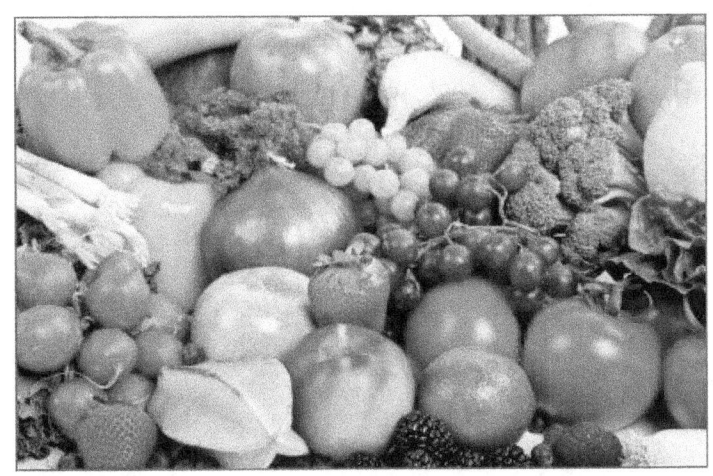

CARLA DENISE

OLDENBERG SHARBONO, M.D.

Other Books by

Carla Denise Sharbono, M.D.

God's Amazing Pharmacy

FOOD IS YOUR BEST MEDICINE

Please direct online inquiries to:

admin@atozpublishinggroup.com or thormahlen46@gmail.com.

For written inquiries:

AtoZ Publishing Group, LLC

40 Plaza Way, 8-132, Mountain Home, AR 72653

Telephone (870) 736-2548   Fax (870) 492-7879

http//www.atozpublishinggroup.com

http//denisesharbono.atozpublishinggroup.com

First AtoZ Printing January 2014

Published in the United States of America

FOOD IS YOUR BEST MEDICINE!

FOOD CAN PREVENT, TREAT AND/OR HEAL MEDICAL DISEASES!

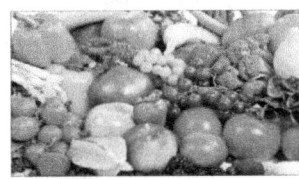

Food is a powerful chemical. Food is as powerful as any medicine. Food can successfully prevent, treat, and in many cases - heal - most of the age-related metabolic diseases, i.e., Diabetes, Arthritis, Obesity, Kidney Disease, Heart Disease, (Hypercholesterolemia / Hypertriglyceridemia), Hypertension, Fibromyalgia, Eye Diseases, Depression, Neurological Diseases and Sleep Disorders, etc. Also, nonnutritive, foods, sweetened by artificial sugars and/or trans-fats can cause these same metabolic diseases.

Also, food can **cause cancer** and food can **prevent cancer.**

Hippocrates once said "Let our food be our Medicine and Let our Medicine be our Food". Hippocrates got it right 2000 years ago.

God's Word (3 John 1 & 2) indicates He provided everything we need for good health: *"Beloved, I pray that in all respects you may prosper and be in good health, just as your soul prospers".*

Contents

PREFACE 1

MEDICAL DISEASES THAT FOODS CAN PREVENT! 11

ABDOMINAL GAS: (ABDOMINAL BLOATING OR DISTENTION):
....11

ACNE: 13

ALLERGIES, (FOOD ALLERGIES): 17

ALZHEIMER'S DISEASE (AD): 18

ANEMIA: 21

ANXIETY: 24

ARTHRITIS: 25

ASTHMA / COPD: 28

ATHEROSCLEROSIS: 30

BRONCHITIS / PNEUMONIA: 34

CANCER: 38

CANDIDIASIS (CHRONIC): 51

CANKER SORES: 53

CARPAL TUNNEL SYNDROME: 54

CATARACTS: 56

CELIAC DISEASE: 58

CERVICAL DYSPLASIA and CERVICAL CANCER: 60

CHOLESTEROL EXCESS: 61

CHRONIC FATIGUE SYNDROME, FIBROMYALGIA,
POLYMYALGIA RHEUMATICA: All 68

COLDS: 76

CONSTIPATION: 81

DEPRESSION: 84

DEMENTIA: 88

DIABETES MELLITUS: 90

DIARRHEA: 94

EAR INFECTION (OTITIS MEDIA): 99

ECZEMA / DERMATITIS: 110

FIBROCYSTIC BREAST DISEASE: 113

FIBROMYALGIA: 115

FOOD ALLERGIES: 115

GALLSTONES: 115

GASTROESOPHAGEAL REFLUX DISEASE: ...116

GINGIVITIS : 120

GLAUCOMA 122

GOUT: 125

HAY FEVER: 128

HEADACHE: 128

HEARTBURN: 133

HEART DISEASE: 133

HEMORRHOIDS: 133

HERPES SIMPLEX: 137

HIGH BLOOD PRESSURE (HYPERTENSION): ...141

HIVES: 145

HYPOGLYCEMIA: 148

IMMUNE SYSTEM DEPRESSION: 152

INSOMNIA / SLEEP DEPRIVATION: 156

IRRITABLE BOWEL SYNDROME: 159

KIDNEY STONES: 164

LEG CRAMPS or RESTLESS LEG SYNDROME: 168

MACULAR DEGENERATION, AGE RELATED: 170

MENOPAUSE: 173

MULTIPLE SCLEROSIS: 177

NON-ULCER DYSPEPSIA: 182

OBESITY: 186

OSTEOPOROSIS and OSTEOARTHRITIS: 200

PEPTIC ULCER DISEASE: 204

PERIODONTAL DISEASE: 208

PROSTATE PROBLEMS: 213

PSORIASIS: 217

RHEUMATOID ARTHRITIS: 226

SEXUAL DISORDERS: 227

THYROID PROBLEMS: 233

URINARY TRACT INFECTION: 235

URTICARIA: 239

VARICOSE VEINS: 240

APPENDIX I: ANTIOXIDANT FOODS.....................................246

APPENDIX II: DETOXIFICATION 248

Biography - Carla Denise Oldenberg Sharbono, M.D. 255

PREFACE

FOOD CAN PREVENT, TREAT AND/OR HEAL MEDICAL DISEASES!

THE MEDICINAL VALUE OF FOOD

I write this book, not only for the millions of Americans who may not be aware of the medicinal value of food but also for those who are "over-weight" and want to lose weight - effectively and safely. Interesting is the fact that most of our modern-day medical problems (diseases) are due to the foods we choose to eat.

 Foods can either cause medical diseases or food can prevent or heal medical diseases. Foods contain nutrients and nutrients are medicinal chemicals. Certain nutrients (medicinal chemicals) are needed by our body and must be supplied on a regular basis from these nutrients in order to obtain and sustain good health. Many processed foods contain preservatives and other foreign, sometimes toxic, chemicals that are harmful and cause many age-related metabolic medical diseases.

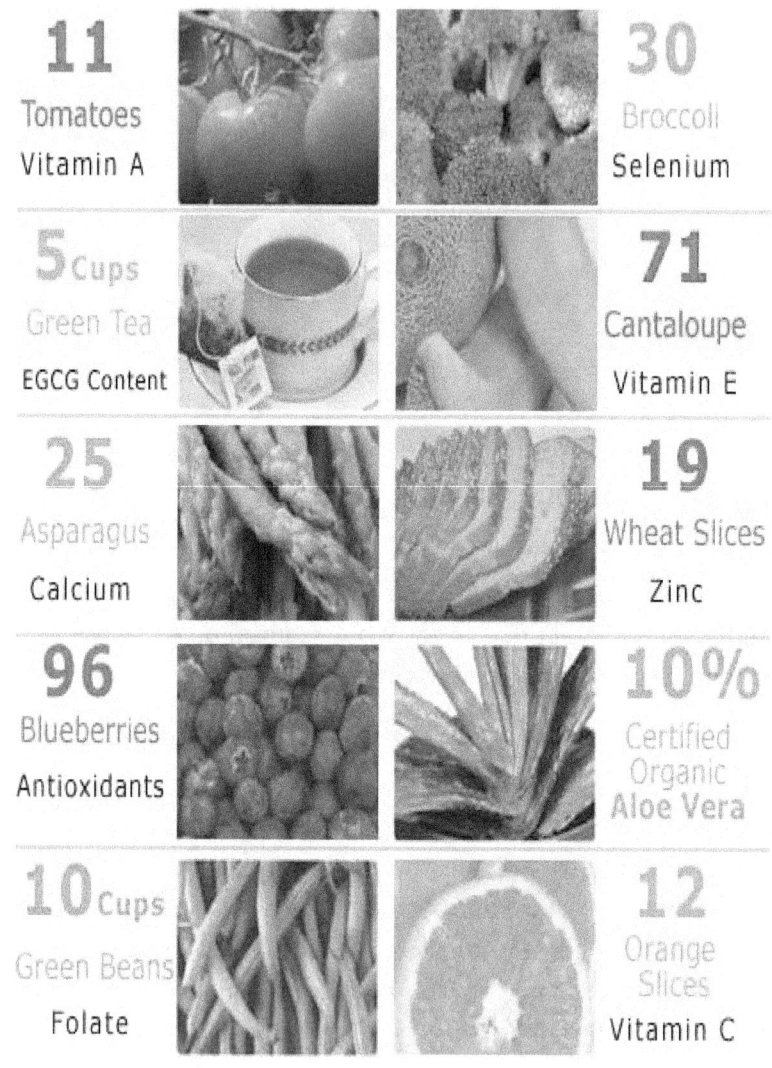

11 Tomatoes Vitamin A

30 Broccoli Selenium

5 Cups Green Tea EGCG Content

71 Cantaloupe Vitamin E

25 Asparagus Calcium

19 Wheat Slices Zinc

96 Blueberries Antioxidants

10% Certified Organic Aloe Vera

10 Cups Green Beans Folate

12 Orange Slices Vitamin C

Nutrients can be divided into macronutrients and micronutrients.

For good health, we require energy-producing, calorie containing macro-nutrients: those nutrients that contain calories, such as proteins, complex carbohydrates and good fats. Our bodies also require the non-caloric (no calories) micronutrients. These non-caloric nutrients are: vitamins, minerals, phytonutrients and water.

Specific nutrients are required for good health and to prevent certain medical diseases. Some of these nutrients are considered organic because they come from living things. They include the nine essential amino acids, (i.e., histidine, isoleucine, leucine, lysine, methionine/cystine, phenylalanine/tyrosine, threonine, tryptophan and valine): the four fat-soluble vitamins, (i.e. A, D, E, and K): the ten water soluble vitamins, (i.e. vitamin C and all of the B vitamins).

The "B" vitamins play a major role in gluconeogensis (the fat-burning process in the liver - that produces energy by converting fat to glucose). *If our body lacks any of these vitamins, especially the B vitamins, we are especially at risk for gaining weight and developing type 2 diabetes , heart disease and hypertension, etc.* These vitamins also play a role in fatty acid synthesis, cholesterol synthesis, choline synthesis and hormone synthesis.

Nutritional oils are also organic and include: olive oil, flax seed oil, corn oil, coconut oil, as well as the omega 3 fatty acids and omega 6 fatty acids.

Some nutrients are considered inorganic. These inorganic nutrients are also necessary for good health. The inorganic nutrients are minerals (mostly metals), electrolytes, and the ultra-trace elements. These must be supplied in the diet - daily - for good health and to prevent medical diseases.

CARLA D. O. SHARBONO, M.D.

Some Sources of Food Nutrients and their function in the body

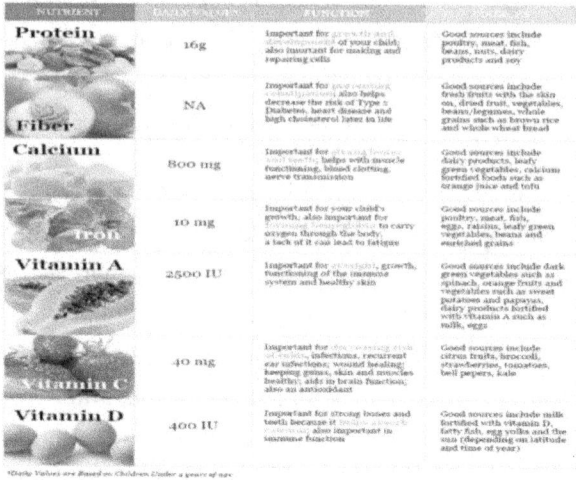

NUTRIENT	DAILY VALUES	FUNCTION	
Protein	16g	Important for growth and development of your child; also important for making and repairing cells	Good sources include poultry, meat, fish, beans, nuts, dairy products and soy
Fiber	NA	Important for proper bowel functioning; also helps decrease the risk of Type 2 Diabetes, heart disease and high cholesterol later in life	Good sources include fresh fruits with the skin on, dried fruit, vegetables, beans/legumes, whole grains such as brown rice and whole wheat bread
Calcium	800 mg	Important for strong bones and teeth; helps with muscle functioning, blood clotting, nerve transmission	Good sources include dairy products, leafy green vegetables, calcium fortified foods such as orange juice and tofu
Iron	10 mg	Important for your child's growth; also important for making hemoglobin to carry oxygen through the body; a lack of it can lead to fatigue	Good sources include poultry, meat, fish, eggs, raisins, leafy green vegetables, beans and enriched grains
Vitamin A	2500 IU	Important for eyesight, growth, functioning of the immune system and healthy skin	Good sources include dark green vegetables such as spinach, orange fruits and vegetables such as sweet potatoes and papayas, dairy products fortified with vitamin A such as milk, eggs
Vitamin C	40 mg	Important for decreasing risk of colds, infections, recurrent ear infections; wound healing; keeping gums, skin and muscles healthy; aids in brain function; also an antioxidant	Good sources include citrus fruits, broccoli, strawberries, tomatoes, bell peppers, kale
Vitamin D	400 IU	Important for strong bones and teeth because it helps to absorb calcium; also important to immune function	Good sources include milk fortified with vitamin D, fatty fish, egg yolks and the sun (depending on latitude and time of year)

*Daily Values are Based on Children Under 4 years of age

Macronutrients are the caloric nutrients. Macronutrients are carbohydrates, proteins, and/or fats. **Carbohydrates** are both simple and complex substances. **Proteins** are made up of amino acid molecules. Essential amino acids are those types of amino acids the body cannot make on its own and nonessential amino acids are those types of amino acids the body can make even if the foods consumed do not contain protein. **Fats** are either unsaturated, i.e., mono, di, or poly-unsaturated or saturated, i.e., tri-glycerides, and transfats. Trans-fats are man-made fats: made by forcing Hydrogen gas into natural vegetables oils (hydrogenation).

Some examples of these hydrogenated oils are margarine and shortening. *(Interesting is the fact that hydrogenated oils are just a few steps away from being a plastic molecule. For example, if you were to burn, at very high temperatures, a stick of margarine it would turn into a glob of plastic.)* Hydrogenated oils are trans-fats and are more likely to cause medical problems than butter or lard, the natural saturated fats.

Cholesterol, a waxy-like substrate, is considered a fat at times. Omega 3 and omega 6 fatty acids are unsaturated good fats as well as many unsaturated oils. Cholesterol is a good fat if it is bonded to the good, high density lipoprotein (HDL). The difference in its character depends on which lipoprotein hooks up to cholesterol and carries it through the blood stream. That difference usually depends on the amount of glucose (sugar) and insulin that are also circulating in the blood stream at that time.

Micronutrients are non-caloric nutrients. Micronutrients are: vitamins, minerals, and/or phytonutrients.

Vitamins are those organic micronutrients that the body cannot make and therefore must be supplied daily from the foods we eat. The following is a complete list of these vitamins. Vitamin A (Retinol or Carotenoids), Vitamins: B1(thiamine), B2(riboflavin), B3(niacin), B5(pantothenic acid), B6(pyridoxine), B7(biotin), B9(folic acid), B12(cyanocobalamine), Vitamins: C (ascorbic acid), D (Ergocalciferol or Cholecalciferal), E (Tocopherol or Tocotrienol), K (Phylloquinone or Menaquinone), and even Vitamin Q (Coenzyme Q10 or CoQ10).

Vitamin Q (CoQ10) is considered a type of vitamin needed to be supplemented by individuals placed on statins, (cholesterol lowering drugs). This is because the body's biochemical machinery for making natural Coenzyme Q-10 is blocked by all "statin" drugs. A list of micronutrients that is recognized as vitamins along with some examples of foods high in these vitamins are:

•Vitamin A (Retinol or Carotenoids), Sweet Potatoes, Spinach, Carrots, Eggs, Fish and Liver

- Vitamins: B1(thiamine), B2(riboflavin), B3(niacin), B5(pantothenic acid), B6(pyridoxine), B7(biotin), B9(folic acid),B12(cyanocobalamine), found in most meats and vegetables.
- Vitamin C (ascorbic acid), Citrus and Non-Citrus Fruit, and Vegetables, i.e., peppers& kale
- Vitamin D (Ergocalciferol or Cholecalciferal), Milk and Milk products, Salmon and Oranges
- Vitamin E (Tocopherol or Tocotrienol), Nuts and Wheat Germ
- Vitamin K (Phylloquinone or Menaquinone), Green leafy veg. - Kale, Beets & Greens
- Vitamin Q (Coenzyme Q10 or CoQ10). A necessary vitamin for strong healthy muscles. A supplement is required if you are taking a statin for lowering cholesterol.

Minerals are elements that the body needs in order to complete, or make happen, the many biochemical processes needed by the body to make structures (i.e. cells, cell membranes, bones, blood, hormones, neurotransmitters, etc.). Some of the most common elements needed by the body are: (1) calcium, (2) chromium, (3) copper, (4) iodine, (5) iron, (6) magnesium, (7) sodium (8) manganese, (9) phosphorus, (10) potassium, (11) selenium, and (12) zinc.

Phytonutrients: phytonutrients are basically the organic nutrient components of plants: e.g., fruits, vegetables, nuts, seeds, legumes, herbs, spices and teas. Phytonutrients are thought to have medicinal properties that promote good health. Scientifically, they are classified as carotenoids, polyphenols (flavonoids and non-flavonoids), indoles, inositols, lignans, etc. All 'food' nutrients are important, but the micronutrients, (especially the phytonutrients), are actually the most important nutrients needed by the body for the maintenance of good health and/or the prevention of most diseases. Phytonutrients contain anti-oxidants that neutralize free radicals and/or they contain anti-inflammatory agents that prevent inflammation and thus heal swollen or damaged cells structures. Phytonutrients are divided into classes. Some of the common classes of phytonutrients include:

•**Carotenoids** have anti-oxidant properties and protect against certain cancers & heart disease.

(1) Alpha-carotene (carrots), prevents eye diseases
(2) Beta-carotene (sweet potato, pumpkin, broccoli), prevents eye diseases
(3) Beta-cryptoxanthin (citrus fruit, peaches, apricots), prevents infections
(4) Lutein (spinach, kale, turnip greens), prevents eye disease
(5) Lycopene (grapefruits, guava, watermelon, tomatoes), prevents heart disease & cancer
(6) Zeaxanthin, (green vegetables and citrus fruits) prevents eye diseases

•**Polyphenols** have anti-oxidant properties and can remove free radicals from the body and anti-inflammatory properties that heal. Polyphenols are either flavonoids or non-flavonoids.

(A) Flavonoids - Polyphenols that have more anti-oxidant properties and are classified further:

(1) Anthocyanin, and procyanidin (citrus fruits) prevents cancers
 (2) Catechins (green tea, chocolate and wine) prevents weight problems and heart disease
 (3) Flavones (fruits, vegetables, tea and wine) prevents heart diseases
 (4) Quercetin (the skins of apples and grapes and red wine, broccoli, kale, onions and certain   nuts and seeds): known specifically to prevent or help fight cancers.
(5) Isoflavones are also known as phytoestrogens (found in soybeans and legumes)
 (6) Isothiocyanates and indoles (onions, kale, broccoli, cabbage, mustard greens)

(7) Sulfides and thiols (onions, leeks and garlic) prevents infections

(8) Rhamnetic (clove oil) prevents inflammatory diseases

(B) Non-flavonoids –Polyphenols have more anti-inflammatory and are:

(1)Ellagic acid (strawberries, blueberries, raspberries, and blackberries).

(2) Resveratrol (a chemical found in the skins of grapes and apples). Resveratrol is an important polyphenol, non-flavonoid phytonutrient that is known to lower the risk of heart disease even though the diet may be high in saturated fat.

(3) Lignans are a group of phytonutrients that are also considered a type of polyphenol. They are also considered as phytoestrogens. Phytoestrogens are estrogen-like chemicals that also act as anti-oxidants. The other classes of phytoestrogens are the isoflavones and coumestans. Sources of lignans include (flax seed, sesame seed, soybeans, cruciferous vegetables such as broccoli or cabbage, and some fruits, particularly apricots and strawberries). Lignans are also good antioxidants: scavenging free radicals. This is an example of natural detoxification.

• **Inositol** is a common phytonutrient that is considered anti- inflammatory:
i.e. cantaloupe, oranges, nuts, bran and seeds.

• **Phenols** are similar to alcohols but aren't classified as alcohols. Examples of phenols are:

(1) Capsaicin (the pungent compound of chili peppers),

(2) Estradiol (the estrogen hormone), found in Borage oil

(3) Eugenol (the main constituent of the
      essential oil of clove),
(4) Serotonin, dopamine, adrenaline,
      noradrenaline (neurotransmitters made from
      protein),
(5) Polyphenol (e.g. flavonoids, lignans and
tannins)
(6) Tyrosine (an amino acid) needed to make
      Dopamine, a neurotransmitter. Found in
cheese,
      turkey.

Phenols are the active constituents of Cannabis, L-DOPA (a
dopamine pro-drug used in the treatment of myasthenia gravis
and Parkinson's disease), Methyl salicylates (a major constituent
of the essential oil of wintergreen), Propofol (a short-acting
intravenous anesthetic agent), and Salicylic acid (a plant hormone
used for its analgesic, antipyretic, and anti-inflammatory
properties, also salicylic acid is a precursor compounds to Aspirin)

<u>Sources of Some Specific Micro-nutrients : i.e. Vitamins, Minerals, and Phytonutrients</u>

COLOR OF FRUIT AND VEGETABLE GROUPS	SOURCES OF ONE OR MORE OF THE FOLLOWING	FOUND IN ONE OR MORE OF THE FOLLOWING FOODS
GREEN		
	Lutein, Zeaxanthin, Indoles, Vitamin K &/Or Potassium	Turnip, Collard, Kale, Spinach, Lettuce, Broccoli, Green peas, Kiwi, Honeydew, Cabbage, Brussels Sprouts, Bok Choy, Arugala, Swiss Chard, Cauliflower, Leafy greens, Watercress, Endive
YELLOW/ORANGE		
	Beta-Carotene, Vitamin A, Bioflavonoids, Vitamin C, &/Or Potassium	Carrots, Sweet potatoes, Pumpkin, Butternut Squash, Cantaloupe, Mangoes, Apricots, Peaches, Oranges, Grapefruit, Lemons, Tangerines, Clementines, Peaches, Papaya, Nectarines, Pears, Pineapple, Yellow Raisins, Yellow Pepper, Bananas
RED		
	Vitamin C &/Or Anthocyanins	Cranberries, Pink grapefruit, Raspberries, Strawberries, Watermelon, Red Cabbage, Red Pepper, Radishes, Tomatoes, Cherries, Beets, Apples, Red Onion, Kidney Beans, Red Beans
BLUE/PURPLE		
	Anthocyanins, Vitamin C, &/Or Phenolics	Blueberries, Blackberries, Purple Grapes, Black Currants, Elderberries, Plums, Prunes, Raisins, Eggplant
WHITE		
	Allium & Allicin	Garlic, Onions, Leeks, Scallions, Chives

MEDICAL DISEASES THAT FOODS CAN PREVENT!

ABDOMINAL GAS: (ABDOMINAL BLOATING OR DISTENTION): Bloating or abdominal gas is commonly caused by intestinal gas. Bloating can be painful, embarrassing, and it can also limit your wardrobe choices to elastic waistbands. Fortunately there are several ways to deal with gas and/or bloating.

Signs and Symptoms: Abdominal pain or tenderness to touch along with an increase in abdominal girth are the classic symptoms of abdominal gas or bloating. Other symptoms include the sensation or feeling your abdomen is tight, swollen or too full.

Causes: One cause of abdominal gas is eating foods that create gas. The best way to prevent gas caused by foods is to avoid those foods that contribute to intestinal gas. Also, swallowing air while eating, often done unconsciously due to eating too fast, may result in frequent belching during or after meals as well as intestinal gas.

To avoid swallowing air, slow down when eating, don't 'slurp' drinks, and don't talk while chewing. Carbonated beverages (such as soda pop), especially when drinking through straws and chewing gum or eating hard candy or greasy foods such as French fries or onion rings, and chocolate milk shakes are examples of more uncommon causes for bloating. Lactose intolerance may also contribute to abdominal bloating. Although uncommon, bloating can be caused by more serious conditions such as IBS (Irritable Bowel Syndrome), Ulcerative colitis and/or Inflammatory Bowel disease. Persistent, severe or painful bloating should be checked out by a doctor right away.

Nutritional factors: Every person is affected by foods differently, but foods that commonly <u>cause gas</u> should be <u>avoided.</u> They are: <u>Processed Wheat products</u>, <u>Asparagus</u>, <u>Broccoli</u>, <u>Brussels sprouts</u>, <u>Cabbage</u>, <u>Cauliflower</u>, <u>Onions</u>, <u>Corn</u>, <u>Potatoes</u>, especially <u>Potato chips</u> and <u>French fries</u>, <u>Milk products</u>, <u>Sorbitol</u> (alcohol sugar), <u>Fructose</u> and <u>Lactose</u> (<u>milk sugar</u>).

Many people are unable to digest lactose, a sugar that is found in milk. This is more common in adults, but some children may also be lactose intolerant. Lactose intolerance is different than a true milk allergy. Avoiding foods with milk, such as ice cream or cheese, can help avoid the problem. Today several products, such as soy or almond milk, are available which are <u>lactose-free</u> and can help those who are lactose-intolerant.

<u>Probiotics</u> have been used to improve flora composition in the digestive tract, a process that effectively reduces intestinal gas associated with abdominal bloating. To reap ample benefits of Probiotics, regularly consume <u>yogurt</u> and <u>kefir</u>, a yogurt-like beverage, that list "live active cultures," such as lactobacillus acidophilus and/or bifidobacterium bifidus, as ingredients.

<u>Whole grains</u> contain all parts of the grain plant, including the germ, endosperm and bran. Because of this, whole grain foods contain more nutrients, fiber and protein than refined grains, such as white flour. Consuming <u>fiber-rich foods</u> can help alleviate bloating associated with constipation.

To attain maximum benefits of whole grain foods, consume breads, cereals, pasta and rice dishes that contain whole grains, such as <u>whole wheat</u>, <u>oats</u>, <u>long-grain brown rice</u>, <u>wild rice</u> or <u>barley</u>, as primary ingredients.

<u>Air-popped popcorn</u> is an example of a whole grain, fiber-rich snack.

Lean Protein: Protein provides amino acids, which your body uses to create lean tissue. Protein-rich foods also promote positive blood sugar levels, brain function and tissue repair. Eat more lean protein foods such as skinless white-meat poultry, egg whites, legumes, tofu, fish and/or low-fat dairy products. These foods can help you meet your nutritional needs while reducing abdominal swelling and fullness.

 Fatty fish, such as salmon, albacore tuna, herring, mackerel, halibut, sardines, lake trout and flounder, also provide omega-3 fatty acids, healthy fats that may help alleviate inflammation in your digestive tract and thus reduce abdominal gas. Legumes, such as beans and lentils, provide a unique blend of protein and fiber, which can help prevent or reduce bloating associated with constipation. For heightened benefits when preparing fish, poultry and tofu, use low-fat cooking techniques, such as baking, broiling, poaching, or grilling in non-stick cooking spray.

 Note: Even though sulfur has many excellent functions in the body, eating too many foods that contain sulfur (egg yolks, bananas, cabbage, onions and garlic, etc.) can cause abdominal gas.

Summary: Whole wheat, oats, long-grain brown rice, wild rice or barley, as primary ingredients of homemade food, air-popped popcorn, as a fiber-rich snack, lean protein foods such as skinless white-meat poultry, egg whites, legumes, tofu, fish and/or low-fat dairy products, fatty fish, such as salmon, albacore tuna, herring, mackerel, halibut, sardines, lake trout and flounder, also provide much needed omega-3 fatty acids, healthy fats, that may help alleviate inflammation in your digestive tract and thus reduce abdominal gas as well as legumes, such as beans and lentils are your best foods for eliminating abdominal gas -"bloating".

 ACNE: Acne is a common skin disorder that occurs in two forms: (1) superficial (acne vulgaris), affecting the hair follicles and oil-secreting glands of the skin and manifesting as blackheads, whiteheads, and inflammation and (2) cystic (acne conglobata), a more severe form, with deep cyst formations filled with pus and subsequent scarring.

Signs and Symptoms: In both forms, the lesions (pimple, blackheads, whiteheads, cysts or boils) occur predominantly on the face and, to a lesser extent, on the back, chest, and shoulders. These areas of the skin have more sebaceous glands that produce sebum, a mixture of oils and waxes that mainly lubricate the skin and prevent the loss of water.

Causes: Acne is most common as well as troublesome at puberty due to increased levels of the male sex hormone <u>testosterone</u>. Although men have higher levels of testosterone than women, during puberty there is an increase of testosterone in both sexes, making girls in this age group just as susceptible to acne. Testosterone causes the sebaceous glands to enlarge and produce more sebum.

Nutritional factors:

<u>Eliminate</u> all

(1) refined carbohydrates (sugar, high fructose corn syrup and white processed flour)

(2) fried foods, especially foods containing trans fatty acids, *such as margarine, shortening, and processed foods containing other synthetically hydrogenated vegetable oils*

(3) oxidized fatty acids *(fried oils)* should also be avoided, as all of these foods may aggravate acne (4) consumption of milk and milk products <u>should be limited</u> due to their potential hormone content

(5) limit milk chocolate due to the amount of sugar and hydrogenated oil that is used in its processing (however, dark

14

chocolate, that has 75% to 80% less hydrogenated oil and more pure chocolate powder, is less offensive)

Specific nutrients: that aid in prevention and/or recovery from severe forms of acne are: chromium, selenium, zinc, Vitamins A and E and foods that contain sulfur: i.e., egg yolks, bananas, cabbage, onions, leeks, scallions, and garlic.

Zinc plays a vital role in the action of many hormones as well as plays a significant role in wound healing, the immune response, and tissue regeneration. Foods rich in zinc are nuts, seeds, whole grains, and legumes.

Also, dietary antioxidants high in Vitamin A and E, such as fruits and vegetables, are important in treating acne because they inhibit the formation of lipid peroxide (oxidized fats).

(Lipid peroxidation refers to the oxidative degradation of lipids. It is the process in which free radicals "steal" electrons from the lipids in cell membranes, resulting in cell damage. This process proceeds by a free radical chain reaction mechanism. It most often affects polyunsaturated fatty acids, because they contain multiple double bonds in between which lie methylene bridges (-CH2-) that possess especially reactive hydrogen ions.

As with any radical reaction, the reaction consists of three major steps: initiation, propagation, and termination.   Initiation is the step in which a fatty acid radical is produced. The most notable initiators in living cells are reactive oxygen species (ROS), such as OH· and (HO2), which combines with a hydrogen atom to make water and a fatty acid radical. Propagation: The fatty acid radical is not a very stable molecule, so it reacts readily with molecular oxygen, thereby creating a peroxyl-fatty acid radical.

This too is an unstable species that reacts with another free fatty acid, producing a different fatty acid radical and a lipid peroxide, or a cyclic peroxide if it had reacted with itself. This cycle continues, as the new fatty acid radical reacts in the same way. Termination: When a radical reacts with a non-radical, it always produces another radical, which is why the process is called a "chain reaction mechanism". The radical reaction stops when two radicals react and produce a non-radical species.

This happens only when the concentration of radical species is high enough for there to be a high probability of collision of two radicals. Living organisms have different molecules that speed up termination by catching free radicals and, therefore, protecting the cell membrane).

One important such antioxidant is vitamin E. Other anti-oxidants made within the body include the enzymes <u>superoxide dismutase</u>, <u>catalase</u>, and <u>peroxidase</u>). <u>Brewer's yeast</u> is also important for healing acne. This is because of the high content of <u>chromium</u> within the brewer's yeast. Onions and Garlic contain Sulfur. <u>Sulfur</u> is considered a <u>natural antibiotic</u>. Eating food rich in sulfur has many health benefits. Sulfur promotes the creation of bile fluid, which is needed for digestion. Sulfur is also known as a natural antibiotic, more specifically as Russian Penicillin.

Sulfur is useful in treating acne as well as other skin infections. Dietary sulfur also promotes healthy skin by helping the body eliminate toxins. Foods that are high in the <u>sulfur-containing amino acids</u>, cysteine and methionine, will also be rich in sulfur.

<u>Warning</u>: A lack of sulfur in the diet has similar results to having a protein deficit. <u>A shortage of sulfur</u> in the diet can result in <u>asthma</u>, <u>arthritis</u>, <u>nerve disorders,</u> and <u>bone disorders</u>. Sulfur can be found in the beta-keratin of nails, skin, and hair. Also, sulfur compounds are vital to the production of the hormone insulin.

On the other hand digesting too much sulfur produces gas. Most of the sulfur you consume comes from proteins. Amino acids are made of sulfur molecules. These sulfur-based amino acids are recycled for making necessary proteins, maintaining tissue health, and forming enzymes. Sulfur can be found in a variety of foods, including eggs, grains, milk, cheese, meats, poultry, fish, nuts and seeds as well as condiments like mustard.

Also, Seafood is one of the best sources of sulfur. Crab is an excellent source of sulfur as well as scallops and boiled lobster. **Summary:** Onions, leeks, scallions, and garlic, nuts, seeds, whole grains, and legumes, fruits and vegetables, Brewer's yeast, eggs, grains, milk, cheese, meats, poultry, fish, nuts and seeds, mustard, seafoods such as crab, scallops, and boiled lobster, veal cutlet, roast beef and boiled chicken, are the best foods to prevent or treat acne.

ALLERGIES, (FOOD ALLERGIES): In theory, any food can cause a food allergy. However, just a handful of foods are to blame for 90% of allergic reactions due to food. If you have a food allergy, your immune system overreacts to that food. All known allergens should also be eliminated, since allergies can weaken the immune system and provide a more hospitable environment for microbials, especially for yeast. Food allergy is more likely to develop in someone who has family members with allergies.

Signs and Symptoms: Symptoms of allergic reactions are generally seen on the skin as hives, itchiness, and swelling of the skin. Gastrointestinal symptoms may include vomiting and diarrhea. Symptoms may occur after you consume even a tiny amount of the food. Respiratory symptoms may accompany skin and gastrointestinal symptoms, but don't usually occur alone. Symptoms of anaphylaxis may include difficulty breathing, dizziness or loss of consciousness.

Causes: The immune system is the body's organized defense mechanism against <u>foreign invaders</u>, particularly infections. Its job is to recognize and react to these foreign substances, which are called <u>antigens</u>. Antigens are substances that are capable of causing the production of <u>antibodies</u>. Antigens may or may not lead to an allergic reaction.

<u>Allergens</u> are certain antigens that cause an allergic reaction and the production of IgE immunoglobulins. <u>The most common food allergens</u> are the proteins in cow's milk, eggs, peanuts, wheat, soy, fish, shellfish and tree nuts. In some food groups, especially tree nuts and seafood, an allergy to one member of a food family may result in the person being allergic to other members of the same group. This is known as cross-reactivity. Crustacean shellfish, (shrimp, crab and lobster) are most likely to cause an allergic reaction. Molluscan shellfish (clams, oysters, scallops, mussels, abalone, etc.) can also cause allergic reactions.

Nutritional factors: *The best way to treat food allergy is to <u>avoid the foods that trigger</u> your allergy.* Always ask about ingredients when eating at restaurants. The United States and some other countries require that eight major food allergens are to be listed in common language, for example, "milk" rather than a scientific or technical term, like "casein." <u>The most common food allergens are the proteins in cow's milk, eggs, peanuts, wheat, fish, shellfish and tree nuts.</u>

ALZHEIMER'S DISEASE (AD): Alzheimer's is the most common form of dementia, a general term for memory loss and other intellectual abilities serious enough to interfere with the activities of daily life (ADLs). Alzheimer's is not a normal part of aging, although the greatest known risk factor is increasing age.

Signs and Symptoms: AD manifests as a <u>progressive deterioration</u> of memory, mental and cognitive functioning and the inability to carry out the activities of daily living.

Causes:

(1) *a <u>reduced level of acetylcholine</u>,* (a key neurotransmitter in the brain that is especially important for memory):

(2) a <u>reduced level of glutathione,</u>

(3) genetic factors,

(4) environmental factors and

(5) the formation of neurofibrillary tangles and plaques (scars) composed of various protein and cellular debris (*<u>toxins</u>*). The result of these toxins is <u>loss of brain cells</u>.

Note: *oxidative damage, *traumatic brain injury, *chronic exposure to aluminum and or silicon (from antacids, antiperspirants, aluminum pots and pans) and *exposure to toxins (chemicals) from environmental sources or burnt oils (fat) from frying: all of which produce scar tissue in the brain, have all been implicated as causative factors. But the most important preventable cause of AD is oxidative damage due to a <u>lack of antioxidants from fruits and vegetables</u>. (See List of **Antioxidant Foods**)

<u>Nutritional factors</u>: Evidence reveals that a lack of <u>folic acid</u> and <u>vitamin B12</u> as well as a lack of antioxidant nutrients and <u>omega-3 fatty acids</u> (especially DHA from fish oils) play major roles in <u>preventing</u> the development and/or progression of AD. Examples of specific nutrients that can be used to prevent or treat AD are: antioxidants such as vitamins C and E, and anti-inflammatory nutrients such as flavonoid-rich fruits.

Mental function is directly related to ones nutritional status, especially in the elderly. So it should make sense that one's diet should **contain lots** of (1) flavonoid-rich fruits (especially citrus and berries), (2) carotene-rich vegetables, such as carrots, yams, and squash, and polyphenol-rich vegetable, such as cabbage, broccoli, kale, turnips, radishes, (3) omega-3 rich cold water fish or fish oil and (4) folic acid and vitamin B12 foods such a dark leafy green vegetables and whole grain foods and/or Brewer's yeast with chromium.

Also, this diet should **limit** (1) sweets (especially high fructose corn syrup and artificial, nonnutritive sweeteners), and (2) hydrogenated oils, i.e., trans-fats like margarine and shortening and processed foods made with hydrogenated oils. Actually, this diet should avoid all highly processed foods, especially those containing non-nutritive (artificial) sweeteners and those containing hydrogenated oils (even ice cream, peanut butter, mayonnaise or miracle whip **if** they contain hydrogenated oils). It would be nice if we could go back to the days when everything was home-made - from scratch (without preservatives and/or highly processed ingredients. Note: Even lard (a saturated fat) in moderation is better than shortening (a trans-fat).

Other Recommendation: Poor detoxification of harmful food nutrients is associated with most neurodegenerative diseases, but especially AD. In particular, research indicates that people with AD have impaired sulfur-oxidation, a process the liver uses to bind sulfur to a toxin to promote its removal from the body. If the sulfur-oxidation process gets "gummed up" or blocked, the body has an impaired ability to clear toxins. These toxins then damage nerve cells, especially if these toxins contain heavy metals or cyanides. Cyanides are naturally found in low doses in apple seeds, cherry pits, spinach, lima beans, almonds.

It is noteworthy that **ginkgo biloba** extract and **acetyl L carnitine** are being investigated for their effects in the prevention of AD. (*Acetyl L carnitine is an amino acid inside cells that transports omega 3 fatty acid molecules to the mitochondria so they can be oxidized "burned" to produce energy as well as transports toxins out of the mitochondria*).

Beef and fish contain the most acetyl L carnitine per gram of any food. **Turmeric,** the spice that contains essential oils and curcumin, an anti-oxidant and the chief component of curry powder and mustard, is also <u>being investigated</u> for its effects in the prevention and treatment of Alzheimer Disease.

Summary: <u>Foods</u> - containing folic acid and vitamin B12 such a dark leafy green vegetables and whole grain foods: Brewer's yeast with chromium: omega-3 fatty acids such as cold water fish or fish oils: flavonoid- rich fruits, especially citrus and berries and carotene-rich vegetables, such as carrots, yams, and squash, and lignans, id est, polyphenol-rich vegetables such as cabbage, broccoli, kale, turnips, and radishes: and foods containing acetyl L caritine, i.e. beef and fish - <u>play a major role in preventing the development and/or progression of AD.</u>

It is noteworthy that ginkgo biloba extract, acetyl L carnitine and turmeric spice are currently being investigated for their effects in the prevention of AD. <u>Beef and fish</u> contain the <u>most acetyl L carnitine</u> per gram of any food. Turmeric, is the spice that contains essential oils and curcumin, an anti-oxidant and the chief component of curry powder and mustard.

ANEMIA: Anemia is a deficiency of circulating <u>red blood cells</u> or a deficiency of the <u>hemoglobin </u>(the iron-containing protein) portion of the red blood cell as well as a deficiency of either iron or any of the "B" vitamins, especially a deficiency of vitamin B 9 (folic acid) and B 12 (cyanocobalamine).

These nutrients are necessary for the bone marrow to make red blood cells. A deficiency of red blood cells or a deficiency of hemoglobin can cause a deficiency in the oxygen carrying capacity of the blood resulting in medical conditions that result from a deficiency of oxygen. For example, anemia causes a deficiency of oxygen to the heart, which can then cause a heart attack. This deficiency of oxygen in the blood stream can also cause a transient ischemic attack (TIA), stroke as well as acidosis, due to a build-up of carbon dioxide.

Signs and Symptoms: include pallor, fatigue, weakness, shortness of breath and even dizziness and chest pain.

Causes: Anemia can be due to: excessive blood loss, excessive red blood cell destruction as in sickle-cell anemia, or a deficient red blood cell production as a result of nutritional deficiencies. Blood tests reveal decreased numbers of red blood cells and/or decreased hemoglobin, and/or serum ferritin (which is serum iron content). Other tests reveal a decreased iron binding capacity and nutritional deficiencies.

Actually a deficiency of several vitamins and minerals can produce anemia, the most common causes are deficiencies are *iron, *vitamin B 12 (cyanocobalamine) and *Vitamin B 9 (folic acid). Iron deficiency is the most common cause of anemia. The diagnosis of iron deficiency can best be made by measuring serum ferritin, the iron storage protein as well as serum iron, total iron-binding capacity, and red blood cell hemoglobin. Dietary iron is important in preventing anemia. Foods such as coffee, tea, egg yolk, Brazil nuts and wheat bran contain substances can inhibit iron absorption thus causing iron deficiency anemia. Overuse of calcium supplements, antacids as well as vitamin B 12 decrease iron absorption.

Vitamin B12 deficiency anemia is most often due to a defect in absorption and not to a dietary lack of vitamin B12. In order for vitamin B12 to be absorbed, it must be liberated from food by hydrochloric acid and bound to a substance known as the intrinsic factor within the small intestine. Lack of intrinsic factor results in a condition known as pernicious anemia and prevents absorption of vitamin B 12.

Note: antacids interfere with the normal absorption of Vitamin B12. This is why B12 injections are recommended rather than ingesting a vitamin B 12 pill. A dietary lack of vitamin B 12 is most often associated with a strict vegetarian diet since vitamin B 12 is found mostly in animals products. Folic acid deficiency can occur when the diet is deficient in leafy green vegetables, beans, whole grains or a genetic defect in the body's ability to activate folic acid.

Nutritional factors: Calf and chicken liver is often recommended for nutrition-related anemia, as it is rich in iron and in all B vitamins. Brewer's yeast (pill or powder) is also an excellent source of iron and B vitamins as well as chromium. Also, green leafy vegetables contain natural fat-soluble chlorophyll as well as other important nutrients, including iron and folic acid.

Other foods rich in iron include dried beans, blackstrap molasses, lean beef, pork, and venison, dried apricots, raisins and other dried fruits, almonds, mangoes, and shell fish. It is important to note that citrus fruits such as oranges and grapefruit or lemons, or vitamin C supplements, have been shown to greatly enhance the absorption of dietary iron and can be used to treat anemia.

Summary: Foods rich in iron and B vitamins such as calf and chicken liver, Brewer's yeast with chromium (pill or powder) are the best foods for preventing and/or treating anemia. Also, green leafy vegetables contain iron and folic acid as well as dried beans, blackstrap molasses, lean beef, pork, and venison, dried apricots, raisins and other dried fruits, almonds, mangoes, and shell fish can be used to prevent and/or treat anemia. It is important to remember that citrus fruits such as oranges, grapefruit, lemons, and/or vitamin C supplements, have been shown to greatly enhance the absorption of dietary iron and can be used to treat anemia.

ANXIETY: Anxiety may be caused by a mental condition, a physical condition, the effects of drugs, or from a combination of these. Anxiety is an unpleasant emotional state ranging from mild unease to intense fear. Anxiety is often accompanied by as variety of physical symptoms. <u>Anxiety, if not treated correctly, may lead to a panic disorder and other more life threatening conditions</u>: i.e. hypertension, an asthma attack, heart palpitations and other heart related disorders including heart attack.

Signs and Symptoms: are mostly related to the chest, such as heart palpitations, throbbing or stabbing pains, a feeling of tightness and inability to take in enough air and a tendency to sigh or hyperventilate. In addition, tension in the back and neck muscles often leads to headaches, back pains and muscle spasm.

Other symptoms can include excessive sweating, dry mouth, dizziness, digestive disturbances, and a constant need to urinate or defecate. Anxious individuals usually have a constant feeling that something bad is going to happen. Inability to relax may lead to difficulty in getting to sleep and to constant waking through the night.

Causes: These symptoms can also be caused by caffeine, amphetamines, i.e. speed, ("Speed" is the street slang for amphetamines when they are not prescribed by a doctor), an overactive thyroid, abnormal heart rhythms, and other heart abnormalities, such as mitral valve prolapsed.

Extreme *stress can definitely trigger anxiety, but so can certain *stimulants, such as caffeine and certain drugs. Anxiety can also be triggered by elevations in *lactic acid levels in the blood due to a lack of oxygen. Lactic acid is the final product in the breakdown of blood sugar (glucose) when there is a lack of oxygen, as in anemia and Chronic Obstructive Pulmonary Disease (COPD). Untreated chronic pain especially severe pain due to a severe burn.

Nutritional factors: There are at least six nutritional factors that may be responsible for triggering anxiety by raising blood lactic acid levels: *caffeine, **sugar,** *deficiency of B vitamins, *deficiency of calcium or magnesium, *food allergies & *excess alcohol.

Summary: The diet should be rich in foods that have high levels of B vitamins, such a leafy vegetables, whole grains, and beans (legumes), brewer's yeast, cauliflower, broccoli, avocados, corn, kale, legumes and lentils as well as foods high in protein such as beef liver, turkey, chicken, duck, lobster, salmon, milk, peanuts and soybeans can prevent anxiety related medical problems. Foods high in magnesium and calcium: such as sea vegetables, leafy green vegetables, sesame seeds, unprocessed meat and all dairy products can also relieve symptoms of anxiety.

ARTHRITIS: Arthritis is classified as one of the rheumatic diseases. Arthritis is a joint disorder due to inflammation. A joint is an area of the body where two different bones meet. A joint's purpose or function is to move the muscles, ligaments and tendons connected to its bones. Arthritis literally means inflammation of one or more joints.

There are many types of arthritis (over 100 identified, and the number is growing). The types range from those related to wear and tear of cartilage (such as osteoarthritis) to those associated with inflammation resulting from an overactive immune system (such as rheumatoid arthritis, an autoimmune disorder).

These are conditions that are different individual illnesses, with differing features, treatments, complications, and prognoses. They are similar in that they have a tendency to affect the joints, muscles, ligaments, cartilage, and tendons, and many have the potential to affect other internal body areas.

Signs and Symptoms: Symptoms of arthritis include pain and limited movement of joints. Joint pain is referred to as arthralgia. It can also be accompanied by red swollen joints such as seen in "Gouty Arthritis". Trauma-related arthritis is related to the risk of injury from specific activities.

Inflammation of the joints from arthritis is characterized by joint stiffness, swelling, redness, and warmth. Tenderness of the inflamed joint can be present. Many of the forms of arthritis, because they are rheumatic diseases, can cause symptoms affecting various organs of the body that do not directly involve the joints. Therefore, symptoms in some patients with certain forms of arthritis can also include <u>fever</u>, gland swelling (<u>swollen lymph nodes</u>), <u>weight loss</u>, <u>fatigue</u>, feeling ill, and even symptoms from abnormalities of organs such as the lungs, heart, or kidneys.

Causes: The causes of arthritis depend on the form of arthritis. Causes include *trauma or injury (leading to osteoarthritis), *metabolic abnormalities (such as gout and pseudogout), *hereditary factors, *the direct and indirect effect of infections (bacterial and viral), and *autoimmune disorders (such as in rheumatoid arthritis and systemic lupus erythematosis). Trauma-related arthritis is related to the risk of injury from specific activities, i.e. "over-use-syndrome".

Nutritional factors: <u>Many remedies for preventing or treating arthritis are found in foods</u>. But some foods play a role in precipitating or exacerbating arthritis. In general, fish oil and olive oils have been shown to have anti-inflammatory properties that can prevent most forms of arthritis.

Many arthritis sufferers benefit from omega-3 fatty acid supplements. Most fruits and vegetables, that are high in vitamin A such as all alpha and beta -carotenoids and/or vitamin C, will also prevent and/or treat the symptoms of arthritis. Most arthritis sufferers benefit from reducing or avoiding (entirely) sweets of any kind artificial or natural sweets and simple carbohydrates.

Gout is a particular type of arthritis that is clearly diet-related. Foods that are high in purines, especially shellfish, red meats, and processed meats such as bologna, can worsen the condition. Certain other foods elevate the levels of uric acid. These include alcohol (especially beer) and those foods containing high amounts of fructose (such as the high fructose corn syrup found in soft drinks). For people with celiac disease, gluten-containing foods (wheat, barley, rye) can worsen joint pain. Research shows that excessive weight and your diet may influence symptoms of certain types of arthritis and related conditions.

The following is a list of foods that may generally relieve arthritis symptoms:

Fruits: especially those that are high in Vitamin C, such as Peaches, Strawberries, Mango Kiwi Fruit, Cantaloupe, Papaya, Oranges, Grapefruit and Apples:

Vegetables: that are high in Vitamin A (beta-carotene), such as Collards, Squash, Sweet potatoes, Broccoli, Spinach, Brussels sprouts, Bell pepper:

Fish: especially those rich in Omega-3 essential fatty acids & high in Vitamin E, such as Salmon, Mackerel, Sardines, Herring, Tuna, Trout: and supplements of Fish Oil.

Unsalted Nuts and Seeds: especially those that contain rich sources of essential fatty acids, (both omega 3 and omega 6), such as Walnuts, Brazil nuts, Almonds, Sunflower seeds, Linseeds, Pumpkin seeds, Grains, all lentils, Chick peas (garbanzo beans), Brown rice, Whole Wheat and Oat Breads.

Turmeric and Cumin Spice. Both are spices in most spice mixtures and cuisines. Cumin seed grows on a delicate plant, similar to fennel. Turmeric, on the other hand is a dried rhizome, the plant bears a similarity to ginger. Both spices have medicinal uses.

Ginger, Garlic, Apples, Fish or Fish-oil can relieve general arthritis symptoms naturally.

Summary: In general avoid sugary sweet tasting foods, especially those that are sweetened with non-nutritive artificial sweeteners, fried foods, milk chocolate, food with preservatives or additives and **trans-fats and processed red meats (hot dogs and lunch meat)**. Eat a variety of natural, unprocessed, foods as listed above.

ASTHMA / COPD: Asthma is an allergic disorder characterized by spasms of the bronchi (the airway tubes), swelling of the mucous lining of the lungs, and excessive production of thick, viscous mucus. The major concern with asthma is that is can lead to respiratory failure which is the inability to breathe: and therefore can cause death.

Signs and Symptoms: Chronic asthma is associated with recurrent attacks of *cough, *shortness of breath, *wheezing and *excessive production of thick mucus.

Causes: Asthma has typically been divided into two major categories: extrinsic and intrinsic. Extrinsic asthma is generally considered an allergic condition, with a characteristic increase in levels of serum IgE (Immunoglobulin E), a class of antibodies found in the serum of most individuals with extrinsic asthma. (*IgE is known as the allergic antibody*).

Intrinsic asthma is associated with a bronchial reaction that is due not to allergy but rather to such factors as: toxic chemicals, cold air, exercise, infection, and emotional upset or Gastroesophageal Reflux Disease (GERD). Both extrinsic and intrinsic factors trigger the release of chemicals, such as histamines, that produce an inflammatory response from mast cells that reside in various body tissues, including the lining of the respiratory passages. Asthma in the U.S. is rising rapidly, mainly due to increased stress on the immune system brought on by greater chemical pollution in the air, water, and the food you consume.

Nutritional factors: Many studies indicate that food allergies play an important role in asthma. Foods that are linked to the production of symptoms of asthma include: eggs, fish, shellfish, hot dogs, processed lunch meats, nuts, peanuts, milk, chocolate, wheat, citrus fruit and food colorings, ordinary tea, chocolate, sugar, greasy foods and even salt.

Some food additives need to be eliminated from the diet, such as *benzoates, *sulfites found in most beers and wine and chlorinated water *tartrazine (FD&C Yellow No. 5) found in most processed foods (mountain dew) and can be found in vitamin preparations and even in anti-asthma prescription drugs (e.g., theophylline),.

The best diet would be a semi-vegan diet. Vegetables, fruits and foods high in omega-3 fatty acid, such as olive oil or fish oil, prevents a buildup of arachidonic acid. In addition, several foods e.g., **onions, garlic, peppers, Brussels sprouts, pineapples** and **all berries** especially **blue berries have anti-asthmatic effects** along **with foods** high in antioxidants.

Vitamin C inhibits bronchial constriction in both normal and asthmatic subjects by normalizing fatty acid metabolism and reducing histamine production. **Vitamin C** is found in peppers, berries, citrus fruit, kiwis, pineapples and green vegetables from the cabbage family.

Also, foods that contain **Vitamin A**, **carotenes** or **lycopene** such as those found in tomatoes, sweet potatoes and green leafy vegetables and **Vitamin E**, found in Wheat germ oil, nuts, seeds, grains, and **Selenium** are also important in reducing asthmatic symptoms. Selenium is found in tuna, cod, beef, chicken, turkey, cottage cheese and Brazil nuts, walnuts and sunflower seeds.

ATHEROSCLEROSIS: ATHEROSCLEROSIS IS THE COMMON CAUSE OF CARDIOVASCULAR DISEASES. It is synonymous with Coronary Heart Disease (CHD) and Coronary Artery Disease (CAD). Atherosclerosis is the process of the hardening of an artery due to the buildup of cholesterol-containing plaque.

Atherosclerosis is responsible for coronary artery (heart) disease (CHD) as well as hypertension (HTN), Myocardial Infarction (MI) i.e., Heart Attack, stroke (CAD) and peripheral vascular disease (PVD).

Signs and Symptoms: Most people with significant atherosclerosis have a history of elevated blood pressure, cholesterol and triglyceride levels, as well as "insulin resistance" whether or not they are diagnosed with diabetes. They may also experience angina (substernal chest pain), diaphoresis (sweating) and/or shortness of breath and/or leg pain. This type of leg pain is known as claudication.

Causes:

(1) Damage to the inner lining of the artery wall mainly from free radicals, i.e., oxidized LDL- cholesterol molecules, is the <u>initial step</u> in the development of atherosclerosis. Atherosclerosis is the infiltration of certain white blood cells (macrophages)and cholesterol (that came from oxidized LDL-cholesterol molecules) that are converted into plaque).

Free radicals are highly reactive toxic chemicals (charged particles) that do a lot of damage to any tissue they contact. Free radicals are produced by processes under-going oxidative chemical reactions as well as produced when foreign chemicals (i.e., artificial sweeteners, toxins, trans-fatty acids) become negatively charged enter the body and are <u>not neutralized</u> by antioxidant food nutrients or the lever cells themselves.

(2) Once the artery lining has been damaged by the oxidized LDL cholesterol molecule, the site of injury attracts cells in the blood (i.e., <u>monocyte</u>s, macrophages and <u>platelets</u>, small blood cells involved in the formation of blood clots).

(3)These blood cells adhere to the damaged area within the artery wall and form what is called "foam cells".

(4) These foam cells then release chemicals that attract <u>triglycerides (body fat)</u> and<u> negatively charged (oxidized) or damaged LDL-cholesterol molecules themselves</u>.

(5) This accumulation of material form deposits of plaque just under the lining of the artery wall and begin the process of blocking the artery.

CARLA D.O. SHARBONO, M.D.

Reducing Risk Factors: The best way to prevent this plaque from forming in the first place is to eliminate or reduce the following major risk factors: (1)reduce elevated cholesterol and triglyceride levels as well as limiting or avoiding both the intake of sweets (simple carbohydrates, sugar & substitutes) and trans-fats, (2)reduce blood sugar (prevent or control diabetes), (3) reduce and control high blood pressure, (4) reduce or stop smoking, (5) reduce and/or prevent obesity and (6) <u>increase</u> the consumption of omega 3 fatty acids and anti-oxidant vegetables and fruits.

Nutritional factors: Dietary steps that will reduce the risk of atherosclerosis include:

- Reduce the amount of highly processed foods that contain hydrogenated oils (trans-fats such as margarine and shortening and processed foods made with these hydrogenated oils).

- Reduce the total animal fat in the diet. Eat more plant foods and cook with olive oil and/or canola oil and even coconut oil, a medium length chain fatty acids.

- Increase your intake of omega-3 oils by eating flaxseed, walnuts and walnut oil, and small amounts of cold-water fish or fish oil - daily. (**Athererosclerosis** - is associated with an <u>excess</u> in saturated fats especially hydrogenated trans-fats and a <u>deficiency</u> in omega-3 fatty acids and medium length chain fatty acids found in coconut oil. Also, it is associated with <u>excess</u> levels of insulin and <u>deficiency</u> of glucagon).

- Increase your intake of <u>heart-healthy monounsaturated fats</u> - by eating more nuts and seeds, including almonds, Brazil nuts, coconut, hazelnuts, macadamia nuts, pecans, pine nuts, pistachios, and sesame and sunflower seeds, and using a mono-unsaturated oil, such as olive or canola oil, for cooking purposes.

Eat five or more servings daily of a combination of <u>vegetables and fruits</u>, especially green, orange, and yellow vegetables: dark colored berries, and citrus fruits. The antioxidant nutrients in these plant foods, such as <u>carotenes, flavonoids, selenium, vitamin C and E,</u> are important in protecting against the development of atherosclerosis.

These foods are also rich in B vitamins, especially Niacin (B3), which can help lower cholesterol (naturally). Niacin also lowers <u>homocysteine</u> levels. [**Homocysteine** *is a <u>bad – (damaging) chemical</u> released in the blood under certain conditions. The amount of homocysteine in the blood <u>indicates how much inflammation</u> (damage) is occurring or has occurred in the blood vessels. It is the best indicator of coronary heart disease and/or atherosclerosis*].

- Increase your intake of fiber. A diet high in fiber has been shown to be protective against atherosclerosis. Dietary fiber, particularly the soluble fiber found in legumes, fruit (pectin), and vegetables (phylum), is effective in lowering cholesterol as well as lowering glucose and insulin levels.

- Limit your intake of refined carbohydrates (sugar, as well as high fructose corn syrup and highly processed refined grains such as white flour). Sugar and other refined carbohydrates are a significant factor in the development of atherosclerosis. Simple carbohydrates (sugar and cookies and even crackers) elevate the level of the hormone 'insulin'.

*(**Insulin** is known as the fat-storing hormone as well as the cholesterol making and/or regulating hormone. Insulin not only increases the body's production of *LDL-cholesterol and *triglycerides, but insulin also raises *blood pressure and *the risk of death from cardiovascular disease).*

BRONCHITIS / PNEUMONIA: <u>Bronchitis</u> is an infection or inflammation of the bronchi, the passageway (air tubes that deliver air to the lungs) from the windpipe (trachea) *into the lung tissue.* Inflammation is your body's reaction to any kind of invasion whether it is from an infective agent or an irritant that produces redness, swelling, mucus, and pain.

There are two types of bronchitis:

<u>Acute bronchitis</u> is caused in most cases by a <u>viral infection</u> and may begin after you develop a cold or sore throat. Acute Bronchitis usually begins with a dry cough. After a few days it progresses to a productive cough, which may be accompanied by fever, fatigue, and headache. The cough may last up to several weeks. If not treated acute bronchitis can progress to pneumonia.

<u>Chronic bronchitis</u> is caused in most cases by <u>exposure to tobacco smoke or other irritants</u>. As a result, the airways produce lots of mucus. Extra mucus and inflammation reduce air flow and cause severe coughing and spitting up of phlegm. Phlegm production and inflammation over many years may lead to permanent lung damage.

<u>Pneumonia</u>, by contrast, is an infection or <u>inflammation of lung tissue: not the airway</u>. Both of these conditions usually follow an upper respiratory tract infection, i.e. common cold, flu or sinus infection and occur more in the winter.

Signs and Symptoms: Bronchitis usually manifests with bouts of productive coughing, shaking, chills, fever, and chest pain that are usually preceded by an upper respiratory tract infection (cold, flu). In addition to these same symptoms, **pneumonia** shows <u>classic signs of lung involvement</u>, including shallow breathing, abnormal breath sounds and sometimes with cough: a chest X-ray shows infiltration of fluid into the lung tissue.

Walking pneumonia, an <u>atypical pneumonia</u>, is an infection caused by Mycoplasma pneumoniae bacterium. Basically, it is not as serious as typical pneumonia caused by typical bacteria. A patient suffering from walking pneumonia does not have to be bedridden or hospitalized. Unlike normal pneumonia, a patient affected by walking pneumonia can move around even when he/she is suffering from this disease.

Although it does not show noticeable symptoms in the initial stage, as time passes by, individuals can experience the following symptoms:

<u>Lethargy</u> or tiredness - sudden decline in energy level. <u>Common Cold</u> - the severity of which will increase with time as the infection reaches the chest. (This differentiates walking pneumonia from common cold.). <u>Sudden chills</u>. Mild to severe <u>headache</u> accompanied by <u>fever</u> and throat problems, such as rashes in throat. Annoying <u>runny nose</u>, <u>Pain</u> in the abdominal region, ears, eyes, muscles and chest. Violent <u>spasmodic cough</u> with very little or no mucus. <u>Sore throat</u> due to cough. *Shallow and rapid breathing due to fatigue. <u>Weakness</u> - which will stay for some days even after all the other symptoms have disappeared.

Prominent symptoms take almost 1-3 weeks to surface. This period is known as incubation period, and it starts with loss in energy levels as a result of which the patient feels exhausted. Before the incubation period, the infection seldom shows any obvious symptoms, and thus mild cases go unnoticed. While walking pneumonia does not make you bedridden, it can be very annoying due to the great deal of discomfort associated with it. It is usually treated mainly with the help of antibiotics.

Walking Pneumonia is contagious. It spreads from an infected patient to a healthy person if the latter's immune system is

35

compromised. Airborne droplets of fluid from the nose and mouth act as the carriers for the Mycoplasma pneumoniae bacteria. In this manner, this disease can spread from one person to another when the affected person coughs, sneezes, laughs or talks. It can strike at any time of the year, but it is most common in late summer and fall - and hence one has to be a bit cautious when it comes to these seasons.

Simple preventive measures, such as exercising regularly, maintaining proper hygiene and eating nutritious foods can help you keep this lung infection at bay. And lastly, it is always best to consult your doctor in case of any symptoms, because any infection, if ignored, has the potential to go out of control.

Causes: both bronchitis and pneumonia can be caused by a variety of viruses and/or bacteria. *Usually these infections follow an insult to or a weakening of the immune system.* Viral infections, cigarette smoke and other noxious fumes, cancer, and/or hospitalization (which increases exposure of organisms that can cause pneumonia), as well as a loss of consciousness, which depresses the gag reflex thus allowing the breathing in (aspiration) of fluids, are all risk factors for these lung infections.

Nutritional factors: *A healthy diet is the best way to have an optimal "strong" immune system.*

This diet should be rich in whole, natural foods, such as <u>fruits,</u> <u>vegetables, grains, beans,</u> <u>seeds,</u> <u>nuts</u> and <u>protein</u> as well as <u>good fats.</u> It should also be <u>low in unhealthy fats</u> (hydrogenated oils 'trans fats' such as margarine and shortening, highly processed mayonnaise and peanut butter) and <u>low in sugar</u> and <u>high fructose corn syrup</u> and totally void of artificial <u>nonnutritive sweeteners.</u>

This diet should also contain adequate amounts of protein. Studies have shown that higher fruit, vegetable, nuts and seed consumption (which are high in zinc and selenium and exert some mild antiviral effects) reduces the risk of developing chronic bronchitis and pneumonia.

Note: **Pineapple**, because it contains the protein digesting enzyme **bromelain**, is one fruit that may help more specifically in the treatment of bronchitis and pneumonia. *Bromelain helps to break down thick mucus and exerts some mild antibiotic effects as well*.

Garlic also has a long history of use as an infection fighter. In fact, garlic has been referred to as "Russian penicillin" to denote its antibacterial properties. Unfortunately, the antimicrobial activity is due to *allicin* found only in raw garlic. This can more pleasantly be done by crushing one clove of garlic and let sit for ten minutes, then mix with a tablespoon of honey to make it more palatable.

Eat one to two cloves daily during any infection. A healthy diet is the best way to have an optimal "strong" immune system. More than just your body's defense against colds, flu and other foreign invaders, your immune system plays an integral role cancer prevention and in vital maintenance functions such as wound healing, repairing broken bones and building new blood vessels.

A variety of nutrients keep your immune system functioning at optimal efficiency. Antioxidant vitamins boost your immune system by neutralizing free radicals, which damage cells and make you more susceptible to infection. Vitamin C exerts antiviral effects even better than interferon -- a molecule released by infected cells that triggers the immune response.

Vitamin A is also essential for optimal immune function: deficiency of this vitamin is associated with impaired immune function and increased risk for infectious disease. Many fruits and vegetables are good sources of antioxidants. Protein: Fish, eggs, lean meats, lean poultry, beans and nuts provide proteins necessary for production of vital immune molecules such as antibodies and cytokines -- immune system messenger cells.

Some proteins protect cells that line the respiratory tract from becoming infected with influenza by holding virus-killing cells (T-lymphocytes) in position along the airways and helping them stay alive and ready to fend off virus attacks.

Healthy fats, such as those in fish oil, olive oil, flaxseed oil and oils in many nuts and seeds build a healthy immune system by modulating inflammation, an important immune component of the immune response. These oils help reduce chronic inflammation, which is associated with increased risk for some degenerative diseases. Fish oil alleviates symptoms of rheumatoid arthritis, an autoimmune condition that attacks the joints and internal organs.

Summary

Your diet should be rich in whole, natural foods, such as fruits, vegetables, grains, beans, seeds, and nuts and protein as well as good fats. This diet provides plenty of zinc and selenium, two minerals known to fight viral infections. Studies have also shown that higher fruit, nuts, seeds and vegetables consumption reduces the risk of developing chronic bronchitis and pneumonia. Also, this diet should be low in unhealthy fats (hydrogenated oils 'trans fats' such as margarine and shortening, highly processed mayonnaise and peanut butter) and low in sugar and high fructose corn syrup and totally void of artificial nonnutritive sweeteners.

CANCER: Cancer is a multifactorial disease in that a myriad of lifestyle, genetic factors, dietary, psychological, and environmental, factors have been shown to either increase or decrease the risk of cancer. And the primary goal should be the prevention of this deadly disease. Cancer prevention is best accomplished by decreasing the controllable risk factors.

However, patients who have already been diagnosed with cancer but who have a <u>higher nutritional load of nutrients</u> are more likely to tolerate cancer therapy and its side-effects: they also have better odds of actually winning the battle against cancer just by reducing the controllable risk factors.

Cancer develops when <u>damage occurs to the genetic code (DNA) of the cell</u>. Cells containing damaged DNA may grow and reproduce out of control. However, most of the time when DNA becomes damaged, the cell can repair itself or that damaged cell simply dies. *When the damaged DNA is not repaired and/or the cell does not die, it will then replicate out of control: and it is at that time these cells become cancerous.*

Cancer or damaged DNA is most often <u>caused by free radicals</u> (highly reactive charged particles). Free radicals can destroy cellular components, i.e., DNA, as well as protein receptors on the cell membranes, and the cell membranes themselves.

Signs and Symptoms: Fatigue, Weakness, Depression, Malnutrition, Digestive system disturbances and other signs of immune system malfunction (infections and sores that won't heal) are just some of the symptoms that the body is fighting cancer. However, nausea and vomiting are among the other troubling signs and complications of cancer and its treatments.

If nothing else is done to control nausea and vomiting, patients may develop anorexia (loss of appetite) and stop eating. When they stop eating a healthy balanced diet, patients gradually lose weight. This weight loss or wasting away, called cachexia, is a sign that the body has started to use up all its energy reserves. After it burns all the energy stored in fat cells, it begins using the energy of protein within muscle cells. Rapid weight loss is one of the most serious signs of trouble for a cancer patient.

Causes: The actual disease process is caused by one or more of the risk factors mentioned above. It begins when the damaged DNA begins to replicate itself and either forms tumors or produces too much of a certain cell type: (as is the case with leukemia, which overtakes the bone marrow's ability to produce the right balance of the other necessary cells for health and life).

However, the cause of most of the symptoms associated with cancer is sometimes the results of "cancer" itself: or are an adverse effect of chemotherapy or radiation. In some cases, tumors produce large amounts of cell proteins called **cytokines** that act on the body by revving up the metabolism. These cytokines cause the body to burn more energy, accelerating tissue breakdown, and speeding up the wasting process of cachexia. Also, it is a well known fact that the many cancer fatalities result not from the disease itself but from malnutrition.

Sugar and cancer: Of the over 4 million cancer patients being treated in the U.S. today, almost none are offered any scientifically guided nutrition therapy other than being told to "just eat good foods." Many cancer patients would have a major improvement in their conditions if they controlled and limited the amount of ingested sugar (simple carbohydrates made from white flour, sugar and even nonnutritive artificial sweeteners).

Glucose (sugar) is the main substance that fuels cancer. By slowing the growth of cancer cells, patients make it possible for their immune systems to catch up to the disease. Controlling one's blood-glucose levels through diet, exercise, supplements, meditation and prescription drugs - when necessary - can be one of the most crucial components to a cancer treatment program.

The saying "Sugar feeds cancer" is simple. Cancer cells have a fundamentally different energy metabolism compared to healthy cells. Malignant tumors frequently exhibit an increase in "anaerobic glycolysis" - a process whereby glucose is used by cancer cells as a fuel with lactic acid as an anaerobic by-product - compared to normal tissues.

The large amount of lactic acid produced by this fermentation of glucose from the cancer cells is then transported to the liver. This conversion of glucose to lactate creates a lower, more acidic PH in cancerous tissues as well as overall physical fatigue from lactic acid build-up. Therefore, larger tumors tend to exhibit a more acidic PH and undergo anaerobic glycolysis.

Cancer therapies should attempt to regulate blood-glucose levels through diet, exercise, medication, supplements and stress reduction. Since cancer cells derive most of their energy from anaerobic glycolysis, the goal is not to eliminate sugars or carbohydrates entirely from the diet but rather to control blood-glucose within a narrow range to help starve the cancer cells and boost immune function.

THINGS YOU CAN DO TO REDUCE YOUR RISK OF GETTING CANCER:

(1) Reduce free-radical formation in your body by - increasing your intake of fruits and vegetables. These foods are rich in antioxidants and anti-inflammatory agents.

(2) Limit your exposure to dietary and environmental sources of free radicals, i.e., cigarette smoke, pollutants and consuming burnt foods, especially burnt fat).

(3) Support your immune system: especially white blood cells. These cells are part of the immune system that circulate throughout the body protecting us against invading organisms. A strong immune system with plenty of the white blood cells is probably the most important factor in reducing your risk of getting cancer.

That is because white blood cells can seek out and destroy cancer cells. These white blood cells can actually gobble up abnormal (foreign) cancer cells. An impaired immune system greatly increases the risk of cancer.

Nutritional factors: Some doctors and nutritionalists believe that cancer is a preventable disease. They say that the various forms of cancer may be caused by bad lifestyle choices, including smoking, lack of exercise and a bad diet. Changing just a small part of your lifestyle can go a long way toward decreasing your risk. A variety of chemicals (nutrients) from plants known as phytochemicals (phytonutrients) also seem to protect cells from harmful compounds in food and in the environment, as well as prevent cell damage and mutations.

It is recognized by the scientific community that there are benefits of eating mostly foods of plant origin. Foods such as **broccoli, berries, and garlic** showed some of the strongest links to cancer prevention. They're low in calories and fat and power-packed with phytochemicals (phytonutrients), i.e., antioxidants that may help reduce your cancer risk. A diet that could ward off cancer really doesn't look that different from the healthy foods you should be eating anyway. That means plenty of fruits and vegetables, as well as whole grains and lean meat or fish is a diet that would help prevent and/or fight many cancers.

Note: Some foods do show cancer-fighting properties, though no one is yet able to say one food or another can stop cancer in its tracks. Still, a body of research suggests an overall healthy diet filled with colorful fruits and vegetables is the key to skirting heart disease, diabetes, and also possibly cancer.

Antioxidants, Phytochemicals (Phytonutrients), and Cancer. You have probably heard of antioxidants, such as vitamin C, lycopene, and beta-carotene, which are in many fruits and vegetables. Studies suggest that people who eat meals that are rich in fruits and vegetables have a lower risk of cancer. Cruciferous vegetables have been shown to help protect against many metabolic diseases including many cancers.

Also, two fruits have recently proven - they can kill cancer cells. Texas researchers have found that extracts from **peaches and plums** killed breast cancer cells, even the most aggressive kinds. Not only did the cancerous cells die, but also no nearby healthy cells were affected. The study suggests that **two polyphenols** (plant-based chemicals) are responsible for the cancer cell deaths. **The phenols are organic compounds that occur specifically in fruits.** These researchers originally studied the anti**oxidants and phytonutrients in plums** and found them to match or **exceed those in the blueberry** — a powerful fruit previously considered superior to other fruits in those categories. Researchers used extracts from two everyday fruits: the "Rich Lady" peach: and the "Black Splendor" plum. The extracts killed even the most aggressive cancer cell, but left normal cells alone, which is very significant.

In regular chemotherapy, normal cells are killed along with cancerous ones, causing major side effects. A closer look determined that two specific phenols — **chlorogenic and neochlorogenic** — were responsible for this targeted kill. Both are very common in fruits, the researchers said, but stone fruits such as plums and peaches have especially high levels of these two phenols.

Besides **Plums, Peaches/Nectarines, Blueberries, and Cruciferous vegetables** the following natural nutrients are also valuable as cancer preventative foods or drink.

1. **Green Tea**. Many doctors and research centers now, including the Mayo Clinic, believe that drinking green tea is one of the best things you can do to improve

your health especially when you have cancer. Green tea contains high levels of antioxidants as well as other cancer fighting agents. Cancer patients who drank 2-10 cups of green tea a day saw improvement in their cancer, and some have seen their cancer go into remission. Interesting to note is that in Japan, the women who oversee the famous 'tea ceremonies' have very low levels of cancer and live to a very old age. This is thought to be because they drink so much tea and green tea is part of their tea consumption. Drinking a few cups of green tea every day may help reduce your risk: it can't hurt and can certainly help.

2. Garlic. In World War II, garlic was used by the Russian army as the **'poor man's penicillin'** when they ran out of penicillin. <u>Garlic has been shown in numerous studies to boost the immune system and to favorably affect many diseases</u>. It has also been shown to improve cancer of the stomach, breast cancer and throat cancer.

The same **sulfur compounds** can also stop "cancer-causing" substances from forming in your body, **speed DNA repair, and kill cancer cells**. Garlic also battles bacteria, including H. pylori (the one connected to some ulcers and stomach cancer), and it has been shown to reduce the risk of colon cancer.

To get the most benefit, peel and chop the cloves and let them sit 15 to 20 minutes before cooking. That activates enzymes and releases the sulfur-containing nutrients that have the most protective effect. And stick with the cloves, not the dietary supplement. Garlic is the powerhouse of the allium family, but onions, leeks, chives, and scallions might also protect against stomach cancer.

Garlic: the protective effects from garlic may arise from its antibacterial properties or from its ability to block the formation of cancer-causing substances, halt the activation of cancer-causing substances, enhance DNA repair, reduce cell proliferation, or prevent the growth of tumor cells in the body. Garlic has been found to especially be helpful in preventing prostate, stomach and colon cancers.

Note: Cook kale with chopped garlic, then drizzle tomato sauce over the dish and serve with rice. This not only tastes good but may help reduce your risk of cancer.

3. Tomatoes and Tomato Products. Tomatoes have been shown to reduce the risk of several forms of cancer because they are **high in lycopene, a cancer fighting agent.** Tomato products such as ketchup, tomato paste and spaghetti sauce have been proven to contain a concentrated level of lycopene, so are particularly good cancer fighting agents. The red hue of tomatoes comes from a phytochemical (phytonutrient) called lycopene, a powerful antioxidant, which is most concentrated in tomatoes.

In laboratory tests, lycopene has stopped several types of cancer cells from growing, including stomach, pancreas, colon, esophagus, mouth, breast, lung, endometrial (in the lining of the uterus), cervical and prostate cancer. Researchers speculate that lycopene protects cells from damage that could lead to cancer by boosting the immune system.

They also suspect lycopene stops the growth of tumors by blocking or interfering with abnormal cell growth, thereby causing these abnormal (cancer) cells to die. Ironically, cooking or processing tomatoes makes the cancer-fighting compounds in tomatoes more available to your body because heat breaks down the plant's cell walls. Want more of this nutrient? Munch on some watermelon, pink grapefruit, or red bell pepper as these fruits are also loaded with lycopene and don't need to be cooked.

4. Papaya. Papaya has a high **Vitamin A and C content and also contains folic acid**, which has minimized cervical dysplasia and other cancers. Some doctors think eating foods like papaya is the reason why even some heavy smokers don't develop lung cancer - this is because of the high levels of Vitamin A and C in papaya.

A wonderful way to eat papaya is chopped up in a fruit salad with other fruits, and covered in plain yogurt. It will fill you up, so is a wonderful healthy meal, yet the calorie count is only around 300 calories for the yogurt and a bowl of fruit. Don't forget though, the best way to improve your health is to combine all these foods with other healthy foods such as nuts, vegetables, juices, seeds etc. Eating a healthy diet will go a long way to making sure you live a long and healthy life. However, these natural cures using foods and drink is not the only important factor.

Note: The most important factor you have to do is to give up the foods known to cause or trigger chemical reactions that cause cancers. Scientists know more about what not to eat, i.e., processed meats, salty foods, sugary drinks, and trans-fats, -- than which fruits and vegetables to pile on your plate.

5. Broccoli. --Broccoli is a Phytonutrient Powerhouse. Remember your mom telling you to eat your broccoli well it is now known this was excellent advice. Broccoli and other cruciferous vegetables such as cabbage, kale, and cauliflower contain phytonutrients called **glucosinolates**, which produce protective enzymes that are released when you chew the raw veggie, rupturing the cell walls.

Your body also produces those enzymes in the intestines, and when raw or cooked broccoli passes through, the intestine, these enzymes are activated. One of the most protective of these enzymes is **sulforaphane**. Broccoli is the best source of this particular nutrient. Scientists believe sulforaphane might reduce cancer risks by detoxifying harmful substances (such as smoke and other environmental pollutants), in the body or by operating as a kind of antimicrobial agent against the bacterium H. pylori.

Broccoli and its cousins are most protective nutrients against cancers of the mouth, esophagus, and stomach. Cooked or eaten raw broccoli contains cancer fighting nutrients. So just steam some broccoli and toss with garlic and olive oil for a healthy dish -but don't add greasy cheese sauce: or just nibble on some raw broccoli florets.

6. Strawberries: are rich in antioxidants. Berries should receive disease-fighting honors. Research points to possible protection against cancer as well as heart disease and memory loss that berries offer. A recent study, using berry extracts of strawberry, blackberry, and raspberry, showed the greatest impact on colon cancer cells by slowing the growth of cancer cells.

Strawberries are rich in antioxidants such as vitamin C and ellagic acid. In laboratory tests, ellagic acid has shown anticancer properties that rev up enzymes, which destroy cancer-causing substances and slow the growth of tumors. They **also contain flavonoids.** Flavonoids are known to suppress (block) an enzyme that damages DNA. This enzyme that flavonoids suppress has been linked to lung cancer. Other types of berries, i.e., raspberries, blackberries, blueberries, and cranberries, are also rich in flavonoids.

Blueberries are packed with anthocyanins, which **reduce inflammation** and are one of the **most powerful antioxidants**. Grapes also contain flavonoids that are well known for both their antioxidant and anti-inflammatory properties. Much like the leafy greens, these anti-oxidants and anti-inflammatory nutrients <u>rid the body of free radicals as well as the inflammatory damage they may have already caused</u>.

Remember, free radicals are unstable molecules that can lead to cell damage and tumors. Grapes also contain resveratrol, which has been found to slow the growth of and prevent prostate cancer and heart disease. <u>Note: Berries and cruciferous vegetables are considered by many to be the most powerful protective foods</u>. Eating fruit, especially berries, probably will decrease the risk of many cancers.

7. Carrots: Carrots are packed with disease-fighting nutrients. <u>**They contain beta-carotene, an antioxidant** type of phytonutrient that scientists believe may protect cell membranes from free radical (toxin) damage</u> and <u>slow the growth of cancer cells</u>. Also, carrots deliver other vitamins and phytonutrients that might guard against cancers of the mouth, esophagus, and stomach. Other studies suggest carrots protect against cervical cancer, perhaps because they supply antioxidants that could battle HPV (human papilloma virus), the major cause of cervical cancer.

Carrots also contain falcarinol a phytonutrient that decreases the risk of developing cancerous tumors. Somewhat surprising, cooked carrots supply more antioxidants than raw. If you're cooking carrots, leave them whole while steaming or boiling, and cut them after they're done. That reduces the loss of nutrients, especially falcarinol, and gives them a sweeter taste as well.

8. Pumpkin. Pumpkin is delicious, and is also known as a super food for fighting cancer. Pumpkins and pumpkin seeds belong to the same family as cantaloupe, watermelon, cucumber, and squash. Pumpkin seeds contain zinc and magnesium as well as a diversity of antioxidants including vitamins C and E. Pumpkin seeds have been shown to fight prostate cancer in men. One of my favorites is to bake pumpkin in the oven for 30 minutes. When it's all soft and mushy, pour a little honey over it and eat. It tastes lovely and is low in fat and calories as well as very healthy.

9. Spinach: A well known super carotenoid source, as it contains an abundance of the antioxidant -**lutein**. Spinach is also rich in zeaxanthin, and carotenoids that can remove unstable molecules called free radicals from your body before they damage it. These nutrients are found in spinach and other dark green leafy vegetables.

Dark leafy greens are part of a class of food known as super-foods. They are filled with antioxidants and carotenoids (such as beta carotene), which help the body get rid of cancer causing toxins. Some studies show they could protect against cancer of the mouth, esophagus, stomach, as well as ovarian, uterine, lung and colorectal cancers. Researchers also think the folate and fiber might reduce the risk of certain cancers, and these nutrients are contained in every dark green leaf.

Note: Folate helps your body produce new cells and repair DNA, and is especially important for women of childbearing age because it can prevent neural tube defects in a developing fetus. You'll get the most micronutrients from raw or lightly cooked spinach. Enjoy it in a salad, steamed, or sautéed with garlic and olive oil, or stirred into soups. For a change, substitute kale, collard greens, Swiss chard, or romaine lettuce. But spinach is the star. Out of the leafy greens, spinach is one of the most nutrient-dense.

10. Whole Grains: especially the ancient grains such as millet, Quinoa (keen-wa), spelt, kamuta, and amaranth, deliver plenty of fiber and contain substances that might battle cancer, such as which act as the antioxidants, **lignans,** and **saponins,** which could keep cancer cells from multiplying.

Always look for bread labeled "100% whole wheat" or "stone ground" rather than simply "wheat bread," which likely contains refined grains. For even more lignans, choose a whole wheat bread sprinkled with flax or sesame seeds. Or choose Ezekiel bread that contains Spelt, Barley, Pinto, Northern and Kidney Beans, Lentils and Millet, Remember, white bread has had most of its nutrients removed.

11. Flaxseeds: are seeds from the flax plant which is normally cultivated for its fiber. The seed, however, contains a high dose of omega-3 fatty acids, which are very beneficial for the prevention of cancer. Flaxseed can be found in many foods such as multigrain breads, cereals and muffins, as it is a compound in most whole grain flour.

12. Protein: Cancer patients often need to increase their intake of protein, especially if they are showing signs of cachexia or are on chemotherapy. Protein is especially important for many of the functions <u>necessary for recovery</u>. It <u>helps maintain muscle mass</u>, <u>nourishes the lining of the gastrointestinal tract</u>, <u>boosts blood counts</u>, <u>heals tissues</u>, and <u>boosts the immune system that helps fight cancer and infections</u>.

Inadequate protein intake slows recovery from any illness and decreases resistance to infection in general. Cancer patients undergoing conventional cancer therapy may require as much as 50% more protein than usual. Smoothies are an ideal – and delicious- way for people with cancer to consume lots of high-quality protein.

Note: The highest-quality protein powder comes from whey, a natural by-product of the cheese-making process. Whey is called a complete protein because it contains all essential and nonessential amino acids. Whey protein has the highest concentrations of branched-chain amino acids and <u>glutamine</u> (an amino acid involved in more metabolic processes than the other amino acids) found in nature.

Glutamine and branched-chain amino acids are critical to cellular health and protein synthesis. Glutamine is especially important as a source of fuel for white blood cells. Glutamine also prevents mouth ulcers (stomatitis) and prevents suppression of the immune system in cancer patients receiving chemotherapy.

Glutamine can also heal peptic ulcers, enhance energy levels, boost immune function and fight infections. Twenty to thirty grams of whey protein concentrate twice a day (or about 40 to 60 grams of protein per day which is higher than the normal RDV of 35 grams) is recommended for those undergoing chemotherapy.

Whey protein concentrate added to water, whole fruit, nonfat milk or soy milk and a few ice cubes blended together in a blender is all that is needed to <u>make a delicious protein shake or smoothie</u>. Soy foods also appear to be helpful in treating most cancers. The possible exception is in women who have estrogen-sensitive breast tumors.

Studies have shown that the isoflavone, genistein, stimulates the growth of estrogen-receptor-positive tumors, but it inhibits the growth of breast cancer cells that lack estrogen receptors as well as most other cancer cells. It appears that for most cancers, especially prostate and lung cancer, increasing the consumption of soy foods offers significant benefits.

Soy foods include tofu (milk-curd) and soy foods that simulate traditional meat and dairy products, such as soy milk, soy hot dogs, soy sausage, and soy cheese. Soy isoflavonoids prevent the formation of new blood vessels, thus preventing tumors from obtaining a blood supply necessary for continued growth as well as preventing tumor cells from dividing and growing by inhibiting enzymes involved in cell replication. Cancer patients should consume at least one serving of soy per day unless you have a history of estrogen-positive breast cancer. Remember, soy milk makes a good base for whey protein smoothies.

CANDIDIASIS (CHRONIC): Candidiasis is a chronic yeast infection. It is a complex medical syndrome attributed to an overgrowth of yeast usually in the gastrointestinal tract. This infection is usually due to a benign yeast or fungus, *Candida albicans*. This condition occurs when there is a malfunction or weakening of the immune system.

Signs and Symptoms: Fatigue, allergies, depression, chemical sensitivities, digestive system disturbances, malnutrition and signs of immune system malfunction are just some of the symptoms of a chronic yeast infection.

Causes: Prolonged use of antibiotics is believed to be the most common factor or cause in the development of chronic *candidiasis*. Antibiotics suppress the normal intestinal bacteria, which strongly promotes the proliferation of yeast. Other factors that predispose to *Candida* over growth are: decreased digestive secretions: impaired immunity: use of other drugs, such as corticosteroids, birth control pills and estrogen pills: and hyperglycemia due to "insulin resistance" and/or uncontrolled diabetes.

Nutritional factors: Several dietary factors do affect the overgrowth of Candida. Number one is food high in sugars. Candida multiplies faster in a high sugar state.
Limit: refined sugar, commercial fruit juices, honey and/or maple syrup. Milk and milk products should be limited due to their high content of lactose (milk sugar). Refined white-flour products should be replaced with whole grains.

Increase: foods that can be eaten fresh or unprocessed include all vegetables, protein sources (legumes, fish, poultry, and meat), and whole grains. One serving of the following low-sugar fruit should be eaten every day.

These include: apples, pears, cherries, blueberries and other berries. Garlic is good for preventing and treating candidiasis because garlic has demonstrated significant antifungal activity against a wide range of fungi. Garlic is more potent than Nystatin (mycostatin), gentian violet, and other reputed antifungal agents.

Summary: for successfully preventing and controlling *Candida albicans*:

- Enhance digestion with the use of digestive aids, if necessary. One simple method is to sip 8 ounces of water with 1 to 2 tablespoons fresh lemon juice or 5 to 15 drops bitter herbs, such as equal amounts of Artemisia and gentian and even dilute vinegar, 15 minutes before meals. If digestion is particularly weak, digestive enzymes (proteases) can be taken with each meal.

- Enhance immune function through high-quality nutrition and if necessary, herbal supplements such as astragalus, Siberian ginseng, and medicinal mushrooms.
- Enhance liver function by eating a high-fiber, low-fat, low-carbohydrate (sugar) diet. **Adding the juice of oranges, cabbage, broccoli and/or carrots will enhance liver function.**
- Use nutritional and herbal supplements that help control against yeast overgrowth and promote a healthy bacterial flora, such as oregano oil, thyme oil, lauric acid, Lactobacillus acidophilus, and Bifidobacteria, i.e., Activia.
- Eliminate Candida toxins by using a water-soluble fiber source, such as guar gum, psyllium seed, or fruit pectin, which can bind to toxins in the gut and promote their excretion.

CANKER SORES: Canker sores (aphthous stomatitis) are single or clustered shallow, painful ulcers found anywhere in the oral cavity. The sores usually resolve in seven to twenty-one days but are recurrent in many people with an impaired (weak) immune system. They are primarily due to allergies and not due to viruses like herpes.

Signs and Symptoms: Finding single or clustered shallow, painful ulcers anywhere in the oral cavity is the most likely sign that canker sores are present. In contrast to cold sores, caused by the herpes-virus, canker sores occur only inside the mouth and are always flat, never creating fluid-filled bumps, or vesicles, like a cold sore.

Causes: Unlike cold sores, which also occur in and around the mouth, canker sores are not caused by a virus. Recurrent canker sores appear to be related to trauma: stress, nutritional deficiencies: food sensitivities, especially milk and gluten sensitivity or food irritants: and/or an impaired immune system response. However, <u>stress</u> is often the most common precipitating factor in recurrent canker sores.

Nutritional factors: A diet that eliminates allergic foods will most often prevent further recurrences. *The most common offending foods are typically <u>wheat based</u>.* Gluten, a grain protein, appears to be major causative factor for many individuals. Also, since the lining of the mouth and throat has a high turnover rate of the cells that line these epithelial surfaces it is often the first place where nutritional deficiencies becomes visible.

<u>Nutrient deficiencies</u> seem to be much more common among recurrent canker sore sufferers than in the general population, *especially deficiencies of Iron, and Vitamins B1 (thiamine), B6 (pyridoxine), B9 (folic acid), B12(Cyanacobalamine).* Foods high in Vitamins B1, B6, B9 are: Brewer's yeast, nuts, and whole grains: *Foods high in Vitamins B12 and B6 as well as iron are: lean meats and fish: *Foods high in folic acid are: legumes and leafy green vegetables.

Summary: Foods high in Iron, and Vitamins B1 (thiamine), B6 (pyridoxine), B9 (folic acid), B12 (Cyanacobalamine) are known to improve the immune system and prevent or treat canker sores. Foods high in these nutrients include: Brewer's yeast, nuts, and whole grains: lean meats and fish: legumes and leafy green vegetables.

CARPAL TUNNEL SYNDROME: Carpal Tunnel Syndrome (CTS) is a common, painful disorder caused by compression of the median nerve, which passes between the bones and ligaments in the wrist.

Signs and Symptoms: Compression of the median nerve in the wrist causes weakness: pain when gripping: and burning, tingling, or aching that may radiate to the forearm and shoulder. Symptoms often become constant and disabling.

Causes: CTS is most frequently caused by repetitive stress or minor injury. This injury occurs most commonly in people who perform repetitive work with their hands (e.g., carpenters, typists and keyboard operators). It can also be caused by serious injuries of the wrist. Basically, CTS can also be caused by anything that produces inflammation or swelling of the tissues of the wrist, such as rheumatoid arthritis.

Nutritional factors: Since 1950, the increased frequency of CTS has paralleled the increased presence of compounds that interfere with vitamin B6 production and its use in the body such as tartrazine (FD&C Yellow No. 5). Tartrazine is added to almost every package food.

Bad Stuff Eliminating foods that contain tartrazine and consuming foods rich in vitamin B6 seems to help reduce the swelling and pain of CTS. Foods rich in vitamin B6 (pyridoxine) include Brewer's yeast, sun-flower seeds, soybeans, walnuts, lentils and other legumes, brown rice, and bananas. During flare-ups, fresh pineapple and pineapple juice, along with fresh ginger and turmeric, may help reduce symptoms due to their anti-inflammatory activity.

Other Recommendations: Curcumin (Turmeric) spice is perhaps nature's most potent anti-inflammatory agent. Curcumin is derived from turmeric (a spice used in the making of mustard) and may be useful in decreasing inflammation of the median nerve, particularly when combined with bromelain (pineapples) and fish oil supplements.

Vitamin B6 (Brewer's yeast, sunflower seeds, soybeans, walnuts, lentils and other legumes, brown rice, and bananas) have been used with some success in the treatment of CTS, especially at a dose of 50 to 100 milligrams one to two times per day for at least twelve weeks along with fish oil at a dose of 2,000 to 3,000 mg once a day (this dosage may be divided into 1,000 mg three times a day with or without food.

CATARACTS: Cataracts are white, opaque blemishes on the normally transparent lens of the eye. Cataracts occur as a result of free-radical or oxidative damage to the protein structure of the lens, similar to the damage that occurs to the protein of egg whites when eggs are heated. Cataracts are the leading cause of impaired vision and blindness in the United States.

Signs and Symptoms: Clouding or opacity in the crystalline lens of the eye occurs in a progressive manner, causing blurred vision at first and then a gradual loss of vision.

Causes: Age is the number one cause of cataracts. This type of cataracts is called age-related (or senile) cataracts. It forms when the normal protective mechanisms of the eye are unable to prevent free-radical damage. The lens, like many other tissues of the body, depends on adequate levels and activities of antioxidant nutrients and enzymes for its normal protective mechanism.

Cataracts form when the lens is either overwhelmed by the demand for antioxidant nutrients or deficient in the supply of antioxidant nutrients and enzymes. Besides age, exposure to cigarette smoke or direct intense sunlight increases the risk of cataracts by creating an increased need for antioxidant nutrients and enzymes in the lens of the eye.

Nutritional factors: Individuals with higher dietary intakes of antioxidant nutrients, particularly vitamins C and E, selenium and "alpha and beta carotenes", have a much lower risk of developing cataracts. To increase your intake of these nutrients, include an assortment of high-antioxidant-containing foods, such as leafy greens, yams, carrots, broccoli, and other highly colored vegetables: fresh fruits, particularly citrus fruits and dark-colored berries: and wheat germ oil for vitamin E. It is also important to avoid salt, foods fried in saturated or hydrogenated oils (trans-fats), rancid foods (especially grain oils and nuts that have been left in an open container), and other sources of free radicals, which are linked to cataract formation.

Particularly important in the prevention of cataracts may be raising glutathione levels *Glutathione is found in very high concentrations in the lens of the eye, where it plays a vital role in maintaining a healthy lens. Glutathione is a small protein composed of three amino acids: cysteine, glutamic acid, and glycine. Glutathione exists in almost every cell of the body.*

The presence of glutathione is required to maintain the normal function of the immune system. It is the master anti-oxidant of the body that aids in free-radical scavenging, immune boosting and detoxification of the body. With low glutathione levels, cells cannot perform many of their functions properly.

Four of the dozens of areas where glutathione is necessary for normal functioning can be summarized as follows:

(1) It is the major antioxidant produced by the body. Antioxidants such as vitamins C or E cannot be made by your body and in fact could not work properly if glutathione were not present.
(2) Our immune systems depend on a steady supply of glutathione. Without it, our immune defenses become weakened.
(3) It is important in detoxifying many substances including heavy metals, breakdown products of cigarettes and automobile exhaust, many cancer-causing agents, and a multitude of pollutants and toxins we encounter on a daily basis.

(4) The major source of energy produced in our cells is derived from tiny structures called mitochondria. These mitochondria would literally be destroyed without the presence of glutathione.

Specifically, in the human eye, glutathione functions as an antioxidant, maintains the structure of the lens proteins, acts in various enzyme systems, and participates in amino acid and mineral transport. Glutathione levels are diminished in virtually all forms of cataracts. To raise glutathione levels, eat plenty of <u>fresh fruits</u> and <u>fresh vegetables</u>, as the glutathione content in these foods is substantially higher than in their cooked counterparts.

<u>Note</u>: **Glutathione deficiency is also a cause of Alzheimers Disease and many cancers.**

Summary: Increase your intake of an assortment of high-antioxidant-containing foods, such as leafy greens, yams, carrots, broccoli, and other highly colored vegetables: fresh fruits, particularly citrus fruits and dark-colored berries: and wheat germ oil for vitamin E. It is also important to avoid salt, foods fried in saturated or hydrogenated oils (trans-fats), rancid foods (especially grain oils and nuts that have been left in an open container), and other sources of free radicals, which are linked to cataract formation. Particularly important in the prevention of cataracts may be raising glutathione. It is worthwhile to supplement the diet with additional antioxidant nutrients. Try taking vitamin C, 1 gram, three times daily: vitamin E, 600 IU per day: selenium, 400 mcg per day: Zinc: and <u>Lutein and Zeaxanthin</u> supplements and plenty of omega 3 fatty acids up to 3000 mg a day.

CELIAC DISEASE: Celiac Disease also known as non-tropical sprue, or celiac sprue, is characterized by malabsorption of nutrients and an abnormal small intestine structure, which reverts to normal after removal of dietary gluten (wheat). The protein gluten and its derivative *gliadin* are found primarily in wheat, oat, barley, rye, spelt, kamut, and triticale grains.

Signs and Symptoms: Symptoms of celiac disease most commonly appear during the first three years of life, after cereals are introduced into the diet. A second peak incidence occurs during the third decade. Symptoms generally involve loose stools or diarrhea, often with fat drops in the toilet showing malabsorption. Other signs of malabsorption include weight loss, the inability to gain weight and failure to thrive.

Causes: The cause of CD seems to be an autoimmune reaction against the lining of the small intestine triggered primarily by gluten. Another major cause of CD is the early introduction of cow's milk. Research has indicated that breast-feeding and therefore delayed administration of cow's milk can prevent CD. CD also appears to have a genetic cause. Cereal grains belonging to the Gramineae family are considered to be the gluten family that causes CD in certain people. The closer a grain's taxonomic (classification) relationship is to wheat the greater its ability to activate CD. Gluten is composed of gliadins and glutenins. It is the gliadin portion has been demonstrated to activate CD.

Nutritional factors: Rice, corn and oats are three grains that do not appear to activate celiac disease because they contain very little gliadin. This is the reason a baby's first food should be rice cereal. Individuals who have CD should begin a gluten-free diet. This diet does not contain any wheat, rye, barley, triticale, spelt, kamut. Buckwheat and millet are often excluded as well. Although buckwheat is not in the grass family and millet appears to be more closely related to rice and corn, they do contain prolamines that are similar to the alpha-gliadin of wheat.

Since most processed foods in the United States contain gliadin, reading labels becomes a must. Glutens-containing grains are often found hidden with wording such as <u>modified food starch</u> found in ice cream, soups, and alcohol, such as beer, wine, vodka, whiskey, and malt. Many gluten-free products are available in natural food stores and on-line catalogs. Other beneficial grains for replacement of gluten-containing grains include amaranth, quinoa, sorghum and a variety of rices, such as brown, red, and wild rice.

Other Recommendations: The protein-digesting enzyme in <u>papaya</u>, papain, has been shown to be able to digest wheat gluten and render it harmless in celiac disease.

CERVICAL DYSPLASIA and CERVICAL CANCER: Cervical Dysplasia and Cervical Cancer have the appearance of abnormal cells on the surface of the cervix. These abnormal cells are detected by a Pap smear. *Cervical dysplasia* is generally regarded as a precancerous lesion: which means these abnormal cells are not cancerous yet, but if left untreated could lead to cancer of the cervix.

Signs and Symptoms: *Cervical dysplasia* does not have any symptoms. Even if these abnormal cells become cancerous there are no symptoms until the late stages of *Cervical cancer*. At that stage there is a malodorous discharge and pain associated with intercourse.

Causes: Recently, attention has focused on the role of the human papilloma-virus (HPV) as the major cause of cervical dysplasia. The risk factors for becoming infected with HPV and developing cervical dysplasia include early age at first intercourse: multiple sex partners: herpes simplex type 2 virus infections: smoking: oral contraceptive pill usage: and many nutritional factors, such as a high fat diet and/or a deficiency of vitamin A and vitamin B9 (folic acid).

Nutritional factors: A high fat diet has been associated with increased risk of *Cervical dysplasia/Cervical cancer*, while _a diet rich in fruits and vegetables offers significant protection against this cancer_. This is probably due to its higher content of vitamin A (beta-carotenes), vitamin C, vitamin B9 (Folic acid) an important nutrient that you get through eating whole grains (especially rice oats and corn), legumes, and leafy green vegetables and fiber.

 Also helpful in fighting HPV and cervical dysplasia are members of the cabbage family of vegetables, including arugula, broccoli, Brussels sprouts, cabbages, bok choy, collards, kale, mustard greens, radishes and turnip greens. In addition to increasing antioxidant defense mechanisms and improving the body's ability to detoxify (glutathione - made by the body from cysteine, glutamate, glycine)and eliminating harmful chemicals and hormones, components in cabbage family vegetables exert direct activity against HPV, cervical dysplasia and cervical cancer.

Specifically, one of the key phytonutrients (chemicals) in cabbage, **indole-3-carbinole**, has been shown to be effective in reversing cervical cancer as dosages of 200 to 400 milligrams per day.

CHOLESTEROL EXCESS: (see also **ATHEROSCLEROSIS**) Cholesterol is a waxy, fatty-like substance in the body that serves several vital roles. Cholesterol's chemical structure is [$C_{27}H_{46}O$]. Cholesterol is an important *building block for various hormones and bile acids: both of which are chemical compounds necessary for many of the biochemical reactions that occur in order to maintain good health and in *stabilizing cell membranes.

Cholesterol is a natural nutrient that the body needs on a regular basis just to stay alive and maintain the daily functions necessary for good health, i.e. cardiovascular functioning, muscle and skeletal movements, nervous system functioning (thinking), hormone production.

Cholesterol, like most every-thing else   in our lives, **is harmful only in excess.** Cholesterol is only contained in the animal foods we consume. (*Plants do not contain cholesterol.* **Cholesterol is made within certain cells** of our body in response to **certain triggers**, such as **elevated insulin** (the higher the insulin level the more cholesterol is made in the liver and released into the blood stream).

There does not seem to be a negative feed-back to stop the cholesterol making enzyme (HMG reductase enzyme). The problem with cholesterol in the blood stream is not so much with the amount of total cholesterol but the type: and the amount of cholesterol attached to the Low-Density-Lipoprotein (LDL) molecule. **All cholesterol molecules are transported in the blood by different lipoprotein molecules.**

 It is the lipoprotein molecules that carry the cholesterol to and from the liver that makes the difference in how cholesterol is used by cells in the body!! *Lipoproteins are complexes of phospholipids and proteins that are essential for the transport of cholesterol, triglycerides, and fat-soluble vitamins. The major categories of lipoproteins are very-low-density lipoprotein (VLDL), low-density lipoprotein (LDL), and high-density lipoprotein (HDL). The lipoproteins responsible for transporting fats (primarily triglycerides and cholesterol) from the liver into the blood stream and then to the body cells are VLDL and LDL.*

These two lipoproteins are associated with an increased risk of developing atherosclerosis only when the LDL-cholesterol is oxidized by free radicals.

This oxidized cholesterol-lipoprotein molecule (LDL) is the main cause of atherosclerosis and is what causes heart attacks and strokes. In contrast, HDL is the good lipoprotein carrying cholesterol back to the liver for removal. HDL-cholesterol is associated with a low risk of heart attack and/or stroke. HDL is responsible for returning unused cholesterol and triglycerides (body fat) <u>back to the liver</u> where this <u>"old" cholesterol is converted into bile</u>: <u>then it is excreted</u> and removed via the bile ducts by the intestines.

Bile is old cholesterol. Bile and the lipoproteins in the small intestine are used to digest or breakdown fatty acids (mostly triglyceride fatty acids) and then aid in the absorption of the mono-glyceride moiety of that dietary fat and the absorption of fat soluble vitamins.

Lipoprotein molecules are made up of smaller protein molecules called: <u>apo-lipoproteins</u>. There are 16 different major apo-lipoproteins. These apolipoproteins are required for the assembly, the structure and the function of all lipoprotein molecules. Apolipoproteins activate enzymes important in the metabolism of lipoproteins: they act as ligands, (keys or <u>attractants</u>) for the purpose of attaching to cell surface receptors.

In fact, it is the "apo" moiety of the lipoprotein that enables cholesterol to attach to its receptor in order to get into a designated cell. ApoA-1 is synthesized in the liver. It is found on virtually all HDL particles. *ApoB-48* is the major structural protein of *chylomicrons*, and **ApoB-100** is the major structural protein of both VLDL and *LDL (the bad ones).* (*Chylomicrons are formed in the intestines by a chemical process that binds phospholipids to five molecules of triglycerides and one molecule of cholesterol, and one molecule of ApoB-48.*)

The triglyceride molecules are hydrolyzed to free fatty acids (removed from the chylomicrons by a lipase enzyme). These free fatty acid molecules (once inside the blood stream) can then be taken into tissues that need fatty acid molecules for instant energy **or** <u>if in excess</u>, these free fatty acid molecules are re-esterified and stored as triglyceride (body fat) in the fat cells. <u>LDL-lipoproteins are</u>

<u>formed in the liver</u> by a process controlled by the HMG-CoA reductase enzyme.

This is the enzyme that can be blocked by "statin" drugs, Niacin (vitamin B3) as well as naringenin, a chemical in grapefruit. The liver also makes another lipoprotein that attaches to the ApoB-100 molecule. It is called <u>apo-lipoprotein(a)</u>, also known as Lp(a). This apo-lipoprotein(a) or Lp(a) is structurally similar to the LDL lipoprotein but contains an additional molecule of an adhesive protein. This protein makes the molecules much stickier and thus more likely to stick to the artery walls and cause damage.

This apo-lipoprotein molecule should be the most talked about molecule when it comes to cholesterol problems associated with heart disease (atherosclerosis). Currently, experts recommend that your <u>Total Blood Cholesterol</u> level (VLDL + LDL + HDL = total cholesterol) should be less than 200 milligrams per deciliter from a fasting blood sample. The <u>HDL-cholesterol </u>level should be greater than 40 milligrams per deciliter. <u>LDL-cholesterol</u> is based on your current health history and risk factors.

Nutritional factors: Circulating cholesterol can be lowered nutritionally by:

(1)decrease absorption of dietary cholesterol through a diet **high in fiber**:

(2) increase excretion of old dietary cholesterol **due to bile and a high fiber diet:**

(3) decrease production of cholesterol within the liver cells by **decreasing the insulin** released from the pancreas. This can be done **by reducing dietary sweets**:

(4) by consuming foods high in anti-oxidants.

Anti-oxidants decrease the formation of atherosclerosis by preventing the oxidation of LDL cholesterol, there-by decreasing the formation of free radicals. Many of the foods we consume daily perform one or more of these actions. *Fiber helps lower cholesterol by binding to bile acids and removing them from the body via the feces. *Fiber also slows down the absorption or transport of sugar into the blood stream which lowers the insulin that will be released.*

Lowering insulin decreases the trigger mechanism for the production of cholesterol within the liver. Fiber comes primarily from whole grains, fruits, vegetables, and legumes. In addition to the fiber components, other grain components help to lower cholesterol. *Rice bran contains gamma-oryzanol, a compound that lowers cholesterol.

Amaranth contains tocotrienol (vitamin E) and squalene (a fatty acid) and Niacin (vitamin B-3): all three are known to **reduce cholesterol synthesis (much like 'statin' drugs)**. Also, diets rich in buckwheat have been linked to lowered risks of developing high cholesterol due to buckwheat's content of hesperidin - a beneficial flavonoid nutrient. Hesperidin is also found in lemons, oranges, grapefruit, apricots, plums and bilberry and vegetables such as green and yellow peppers and broccoli.

Anthocyanin is a flavonoid found in sorghum. These nutrients are all powerful antioxidant that exhibits potent free radical scavenging activity that is known to decrease the oxidation of LDL-cholesterol and thus decrease atherosclerosis from building up within the artery lining. Eat a variety of fruits for their antioxidant effects as well as soluble fiber.

Pectin is a soluble fiber that can help lower cholesterol levels through decreasing both absorption and decreasing the synthesis of cholesterol. Pectin is found in apples, grapefruit, oranges and pear. (Whole fruit contain more pectin than fruit juice unless the skins are included in the juice). Dates contain the soluble fiber – beta-D-glucan. Prunes contain large amounts of phenolic compounds, which inhibit free-radical damage and thus inhibit the oxidation of LDL-cholesterol. Olives and olive oil contains antioxidants, including oleuropreins and flavonoids that act to protect against oxidative damage to the LDL (lipoprotein).

 Fried foods become oxidized fatty acids and have been linked to high levels of damaged LDL (lipoprotein) and the accumulation of cholesterol from LDL within artery walls. When attempting to lower cholesterol through diet, it is important to eat a variety of cholesterol-lowering vegetables, such as beets, celery, eggplant, garlic and onion, peppers and root vegetables like turnips and carrots and yams.

 Also, dandelion root and Jerusalem artichoke contain the fiber inulin, which improves production of antioxidant enzymes while decreasing total cholesterol and triglyceride levels and raising concentrations of beneficial HDL cholesterol. Eat plenty of chili peppers. They contain substances that have been shown to prevent clot formation, reduce blood cholesterol and triglyceride levels and reduce platelet aggregation.

Nutrients in peppers (especially chili peppers) reduce the risk of atherosclerosis build-up and therefore reduce the risk of heart attacks and strokes. Diets rich in legumes, such as peanuts, and soy protein can be used to lower cholesterol levels. Nuts and seeds, particularly almonds and walnuts, are useful in lowering cholesterol through their fiber, mono-unsaturated oil, and their essential fatty acid content.

Hazelnuts have a very high concentration of **copper**, a key component in the intracellular antioxidant _superoxide dismutase_, which disarms free radicals before they oxidize (damage)LDL-cholesterol and triglycerides. Ground flaxseed, avocados, cocoa butter, brewer's yeast, royal jelly, shiitake mushrooms, saffron, turmeric, honey, shellfish and alfalfa sprouts lower the apolipoprotein B-100 ligand of the LDL (lipoproteins) molecule that is attached to the sticky adhesive protein [Lp(a) lipoproteins]. Lp(a) is the lipoprotein that is structurally like LDL. It is the sticky protein that makes the LDL-cholesterol molecule much more likely to stick to the artery walls and cause damage. Milk fat also contains a number of bioactive components, including conjugated linoleic acid (CLA).

Conjugated linoleic acid (an omega-6 fatty acid molecule) has been shown to possess activities that prevent cancer and the formation of cholesterol-containing plaques that contribute to heart disease. Cheese provides many of the same nutritional benefits and health benefits attributed to milk, and it usually contains beneficial bacteria that produce propionic acid, which nourishes the cells of the colon and lowers blood cholesterol levels. It is now known that niacin does much more than lower total cholesterol.

Specifically, niacin has been shown to lower LDL cholesterol, Lp(a) lipoprotein, triglyceride, and fibrinogen levels while simultaneously raising HDL cholesterol levels. Despite the fact that niacin has demonstrated better overall results in reducing risk factors for coronary heart disease than other cholesterol-lowering pharmaceutical agents, physicians are often reluctant to prescribe niacin.

No pharmaceutical company stands to earn the huge profits that the other lipid-lowering agents have generated.

As a result, niacin does not benefit from the intensive advertising that focuses upon the **"statin" drugs.** Several studies have compared niacin to approved cholesterol lowering drugs (i.e. "statins"). These studies have shown significant advantages for niacin (B3). The percentage increase in HDL-cholesterol was also dramatically in favor of niacin. Equally as impressive was the percentage decrease in Lp(a) lipoprotein levels due to niacin.

Niacin along with a low carbohydrate, healthy fats and high protein diet is recommended for lowering cholesterol along with increased physical activity. Naringenin is a flavanone, a type of flavonoid polyphenol that is considered to have a bioactive effect on human health as an antioxidant, an anti-inflammatory, a carbohydrate and cholesterol metabolism promoter, immune system modulator. Naringenin is the predominant flavanone in grapefruit, oranges, and even tomato skins and increases statin drugs level to become toxic to the liver.

CHRONIC FATIGUE SYNDROME, FIBROMYALGIA, POLYMYALGIA RHEUMATICA: All are common names used to designate a significantly debilitating medical disorder or group of disorders generally defined by persistent fatigue and even pain, accompanied by other specific symptoms for a minimum of six months, not due to ongoing exertion, not substantially relieved by rest, nor caused by other medical conditions. These disorder may also be referred to as chronic fatigue syndrome (CFS), polymyalgia rheumatica (PMR), fibromyalgia or post-viral fatigue syndrome.

Signs and Symptoms of CFS include post-exertional malaise, unrefreshing sleep, widespread muscle and joint pain, sore throat, headaches of a type not previously experienced, cognitive (thinking and/or memory) difficulties, chronic, often severe, mental and physical exhaustion, and other characteristic symptoms in a previously healthy and active person.

Persons with CFS may report additional symptoms including muscle weakness, increased sensitivity to light, sounds and smells, orthostatic intolerance, digestive disturbances, depression, and cardiac and respiratory problems. It is unclear if these symptoms represent co-morbid conditions or are produced by an underlying etiology of CFS.

CFS symptoms vary from person to person in number, type, and severity. CFS occurs more often in women than men, and is less prevalent among children and adolescents. The quality of life is particularly and uniquely disrupted in CFS. There is agreement in the medical community on the genuine threat to health, happiness and productivity posed by CFS.

However, various physicians' groups, researchers and patient advocates promote different nomenclature, diagnostic criteria, etiologic hypotheses and treatments, resulting in controversy about many aspects of the disorder. The name "chronic fatigue syndrome" itself is controversial as many patients and advocacy groups believe the name trivializes the medical condition and want the name changed.

Causes: Biological, genetic, infectious and psychological mechanisms have been proposed for the development and persistence of symptoms but the etiology of CFS is not fully understood and may have multiple causes. Note: There is no diagnostic laboratory test or biomarker for CFS. The majority of CFS cases start suddenly, and are usually accompanied by a "flu-like illness".

However, a significant proportion of cases begin within several months of severe adverse stress. Then too, accurate reporting of the prevalence and exact roles of infection and stress in the development of CFS are currently unknown.

The CDC recommends the following three criteria be fulfilled in order for a person to receive the diagnosis of CFS: (1) A new onset (not lifelong) of severe fatigue for six consecutive months or greater duration which is unrelated to exertion, and is not substantially relieved by rest, and is not a result of other medical conditions. (2) The fatigue causes a significant reduction of previous activity levels. (3) Four or more of the following symptoms that last six months or longer are:

1. Impaired memory or concentration.

2. Post-exertional malaise, where physical or mental exertions bring on "extreme, prolonged exhaustion and sickness".

3. Unrefreshing sleep,

4. Muscle pain (myalgia),

5. Pain in multiple joints (arthralgia),

6. Headaches of a new kind or greater severity,

7. Sore throat and frequent or recurring tender lymph nodes (cervical or axillary).

8. Other common symptoms include: Irritable bowel, abdominal pain, nausea, diarrhea or bloating, Chills and night sweats, Brain fog, Chest pain, Shortness of breath, Chronic cough, Visual disturbances (blurring, sensitivity to light, eye pain or dry eyes), Allergies or sensitivities to foods, alcohol, odors, chemicals, medications or noise, Difficulty maintaining upright position (orthostatic instability, irregular heartbeat, dizziness, balance problems or fainting),

9. Psychological problems (depression, irritability, mood swings, anxiety, panic attacks).

The CDC proposes that persons with symptoms resembling those of CFS consult a physician to rule out several treatable illnesses: i.e., Lyme disease, sleep disorders, depression, alcohol/substance abuse, diabetes, hypothyroidism, mononucleosis (mono), lupus, multiple sclerosis (MS), chronic hepatitis and various malignancies.

Interesting to note is that medications can also cause side effects that mimic symptoms of CFS.

Other factors: All ethnic and racial groups appear susceptible to the illness, but lower income groups are slightly more likely to develop CFS. More women than men get CFS: between 60 and 85% of cases are women. However, there is some indication that the prevalence of CFS among men is underreported. The illness is reported to occur more frequently in people between the ages of 40 and 59. CFS is less prevalent among children and adolescents than adults. Blood relatives of people who have CFS appear to be more predisposed. There is no direct evidence that CFS is contagious, though it is seen in members of the same family: this is believed to be a familial or genetic link but more research is required for a definitive answer.

Differential diagnoses. Certain medical conditions can cause many symptoms of CFS and must be ruled out before a diagnosis of CFS can be given. These conditions include: anemia, hypothyroidism, diabetes and certain psychiatric disorders just to mention a few of the diseases that must be ruled out if the patient presents with appropriate symptoms. People with fibromyalgia (FM, or fibromyalgia syndrome, FMS) present only with muscle pain and sleep disturbances.

Fatigue and muscle pain occurs frequently in the initial phase of various hereditary muscle disorders and in several autoimmune, endocrine and metabolic syndromes: and are frequently labeled as CFS or fibromyalgia in the absence of obvious biochemical or metabolic abnormalities and neurological symptoms. Multiple chemical sensitivities, the Gulf War syndrome and the post-polio syndrome have symptoms similar to those of CFS, and the last, post-polio syndrome is also theorized to have a common pathophysiology.

Depressive symptoms seen in CFS may be differentially diagnosed from primary depression due to the absence of anhedonia and labile indifference. The presence of somatic symptoms such as sore throat, swollen lymph nodes, and exercise intolerance with post-exertional exacerbation of symptoms are more associated with depression seen in CFS patients. Many CFS patients will also have, or appear to have, other medical problems or related diagnoses.

Co-morbid fibromyalgia is common, where only patients with fibromyalgia show abnormal pain responses. Fibromyalgia occurs in a large percentage of CFS patients between onset and the second year, and because of this some researchers suggest fibromyalgia and CFS are related. As previously mentioned, many CFS sufferers also experience symptoms of irritable bowel syndrome, tempero-mandibular joint (TMJ) pain, headache including migraines, and other forms of myalgia.

CFS patients have significantly higher rates of current mood disorders than the general population. Feeling depressed is also a commonplace reaction to the losses caused by chronic illness which can in some cases become a co-morbid situational depression. CFS is significantly more common in women with endometriosis compared with women in the general USA population.

The disorder we call chronic fatigue syndrome (CFS) does not appear to be new. The current interest in attempting to define and treat it stems from several studies in the mid-1980s that found elevated levels of antibody to Epstein-Barr virus in people with CFS-like symptoms. Most of these individuals had a history of infectious mononucleosis a few years earlier.

Factors Suspected of Promoting or Triggering Chronic Fatigue Syndrome are: Hypoxemia (low blood oxygen), Endocrine (hormone) dysfunction, Immune (infection) dysfunction, Stress-related disorders, and Somatoform disorder, Viral infections and Nutritional deficiencies.

Nutritional factors: _Studies suggest a number of nutritional deficiencies may have etiologic relevance. These include **deficiencies of various phytonutrients**, especially Vitamins B and C and Q (coenzyme Q10), L-tryptophan (essential amino-acid), acetyl-L-carnitine (a non-essential amino-acid), magnesium, zinc, sodium, and essential fatty acids. Any of these nutrients could be marginally deficient in CFS patients, a finding that appears to be due to the illness process as well as to inadequate diets. It is likely that marginal deficiencies not only contribute to the clinical manifestations of the syndrome, but also are detrimental to the healing processes.

Folic acid: A subset of CFS patients appears to be deficient in folic acid. What makes this finding particularly interesting is the fact that serum folate is highly correlated with the folate level of the cerebrospinal fluid. Although the brain maintains adequate folate levels longer than most tissues, a chronically low serum folic acid level - and thus a chronically low cerebrospinal fluid folic acid level - would be a reasonable basis for suspecting that brain folate could be diminished in CFS, causing impairment in brain function. Note: Folic acid is important for normal brain function. Fatigue and depression, common findings in CFS, are also prominent features of folate deficiency. Moreover, several experimental studies found folate supplementation to be effective for improving mood in folate-deficient members of the general population. A folate deficiency can also cause depression.

Vitamin B12: As in the case of folic acid deficiency, fatigue and depression are features that also suggest a B12 deficiency and could contribute to the clinical picture in a subset of patients. There is data supporting the theory that vitamin B12, given by injection or now by formulations allowing sublingual B12 delivery, is therapeutic. An accepted regimen for treating <u>vitamin B12 deficiency</u> is to initially administer 1000 mcg (IM) of the vitamin weekly.

The patient usually responds rapidly, and the dose is then decreased to 1000 mcg each month for as long as needed. The vitamin injections results in a significant increase in feelings of well-being. A substantial amount of vitamin B12 appears to be necessary to relieve the symptoms of CFS, compared to the amount needed to correct a B12 deficiency in general: thus, the vitamin appears to exert a pharmacologic effect. As a drug,<u> vitamin B12 seems to also have substantial **analgesic (pain) relieving** </u>properties. Other "B" vitamins for which there is evidence of a deficiency in CFS include: riboflavin (B2), thiamine (B1), and pyridoxine (B6). While niacin (B3) deficiency in this disorder has not been studied, there is evidence that supplementation with food nutrients rich in niacin are helpful in relieving symptoms also.

Vitamin C: Depression is the first symptom of scurvy, and a marginal deficiency of vitamin C may cause fatigue, lassitude, and depression which responds to supplementation. Like vitamin B12, <u>ascorbic acid (vitamin C) appears to exert a substantial **analgesic effect** at pharmacologic dosages</u> (3,000 to 10,000 mg daily). In a double-blind crossover study, supplementation of normal volunteers with 1 gm vitamin C three times daily reduced delayed-onset muscle soreness following strenuous exercise.

One study showed: severely ill cancer patients receiving 10 grams daily experienced a significant reduction in pain. Vitamin C supplementation also bolsters immune responses. In persons with recurrent infections due to primary defects of phagocytic function, vitamin C is considered to be the specific therapy. (*Phagocytes are white blood cells that 'eat' invading bacteria and dead or dying cells such as those infected by viruses and attacked by other immune cells).* Vitamin C has considerable antiviral activity which may be due, at least in part, to enhanced interferon activity.

Magnesium is an important mineral for muscle strength. Stress hormones, including both catecholamines and corticosteroids, require magnesium. Many of the symptoms and findings in CFS resemble those of magnesium deficiency. Some subjective findings of magnesium deficiency include: psychiatric and neuromuscular disorders, i.e., weakness, paresthesias, depression, anxiety, sleep disturbances, migraine & tension headaches.

Objective findings of magnesium deficiency are - EEG abnormalities, electromyographic abnormalities, sensorineural abnormalities, and immunologic disorders. Among CFS patients seen in clinical settings, magnesium deficiency appears to be common. Many CFS patients who are magnesium-deficient could possibly derive benefit from magnesium supplementation: particularly when fibromyalgia is a substantial component of the clinical picture. Magnesium therapy for fatigue may take two weeks for a good response.

Sodium is another important mineral. Neurally-mediated hypotension due to hyponatremia has now been identified as a common finding in chronic fatigue syndrome. This syndrome is associated with a sodium deficiency. Symptoms associated with inadequate sodium intake also include undue fatigue after moderate exertion, lassitude, headache, sleeplessness, and inability to concentrate: this symptom complex has even been reproduced with experimental salt restriction. The ability of sodium intake to affect blood pressure regulation through its effect on blood volume is well known, suggesting this subgroup of CFS patients may benefit by moderately increasing their salt intake.

Zinc is another mineral often marginally deficient in CFS. It is interesting that zinc deficiency can cause muscle pain, risk of viral infections and fatigue. Note: extracellular zinc levels have been reported to influence the twitch-tension relationship in muscle, presumably due to a direct effect at the level of the cellular membrane. Leukonychia, a term referring to white spots on the fingernails, is believed to be a sign of marginal zinc deficiency and has been found to be correlated with frequent feelings of drowsiness and fatigue.

COLDS: The common cold (also known as nasopharyngitis, rhinopharyngitis, acute coryza, or a cold) is a viral infectious disease of the upper respiratory system which affects primarily the nose. Symptoms include a cough, sore throat, runny nose, and fever which usually resolve in seven to ten days, with some symptoms lasting up to three weeks. Well over 200 viruses are implicated in the cause of the common cold: the rhinoviruses are the most common. Upper respiratory tract infections are loosely divided by the areas they affect, with the common cold primarily affecting the nose, the throat (pharyngitis), and the sinuses (sinusitis).

The primary method of prevention is by hand washing with some evidence to support the effectiveness of wearing face masks. No cure for the common cold exists. Symptoms can be treated with both OTC medication and nutritious food. However, the common cold can be prevented by a healthy immune system and reducing exposure to these viruses. It is the most frequent infectious disease in humans with the average adult contracting two to three colds a year and the average child contracting between six and twelve.

Signs and Symptoms: Runny nose is the most common symptom of the common cold with fever and headache being next and cough due to post nasal drip being third. These symptoms are mostly due to the body's immune response to the infection rather than to tissue destruction by the viruses themselves.

Causes: The cause is due to a viral infection of the upper respiratory system. These infections have been with humanity since antiquity.

Nutritional factors: Certain foods can help prevent colds and provide some relief from symptoms. There is no better way to bolster your immune system than by incorporating at least <u>five servings of fruits and vegetables into your daily diet</u>.

A strong immune system could stave off a cold from striking you in the first place. And it certainly will give you more ability to fight the colds you do catch. Forget Crash Dieting. Losing more than one pound a week by dieting can suppress the function of one type of immune cells, namely the T-cells. T-cells are white blood cells that target and kill microbes and microbe-infected cells. Researchers noted that the suppression of T-cell production was only temporary, but still caution against losing more than a pound a week on a diet.

<u>Foods that are believed to work best </u>when you are fighting a cold or trying to avoid getting sick are: <u>Passion Fruits</u> like guavas melons and papaya and pineapple: they helps soothe a sore throat and more. And, ounce for ounce, guavas, which are similar to melons, have triple the vitamin C of oranges. However, oranges are still a great alternative for providing vitamin C and boosting the immune system.

<u>Vitamin A</u> has been shown to improve the disease-fighting ability of skin and mucous membranes and is necessary for production and activity of several types of white blood cells. *The best food sources are green and yellow vegetables, including carrots (raw are better than cooked), spinach and winter squash.* Spice Up Your Life.

Consume something with a little zing, especially foods made with <u>chili peppers, hot mustard, or horseradish</u>, to help <u>clear congestion</u>. Get <u>Plenty of Fluids</u>. The reason is the liquid keeps mucous membranes moist, enabling them to trap cold viruses and dispose of them before they can infect more of your cells. The most recommended fluid is water, but also diluted fruit juices, alka-seltzer, decaffeinated tea and coffee. Aim for eight glasses a day. Drinking enough fluids is especially important in the winter when indoor and outdoor air is much drier.

Forget Alcohol. The one fluid you definitely want to avoid when sick with a cold is alcohol. Several studies indicate that alcohol seems to impair the immune system's ability to wipe out cells infected with the cold virus. It is best to save that beer or glass of wine for days when you are feeling well.

Zinc: No cold remedy has gotten more attention in the past few years than the mineral zinc. According to studies, zinc blocks the cold virus's ability to adhere to the lining of the respiratory tract. To achieve the desired effect from the zinc, you need to take one lozenge every two to three hours while you are awake. If you prefer, instead of the lozenges, you could try *increasing the amount of zinc-rich foods in your diet. Steak, pork, crab, wheat germ, brown rice and oatmeal are high in zinc.*

Warm Salt Water helps relieve some symptoms. Gargling with an 8-ounce glass of warm water and a few teaspoons of salt makes a sore throat feel better and drains clogged sinuses. You need to gargle at least three times a day.

Tea: Tea contains theophylline, a natural substance that opens up congested air spaces and helps drain upper-respiratory passages. The warmth of the tea also soothes a sore throat. A little honey can help stimulate mucus production and reduce the throat tickle that accompanies many colds. There are a few herbs that might prove helpful.

Echinacea: This daisy-like herb has its share of believers and doubters. Those who swear by it believe that Echinacea contains substances capable of strengthening the immune system and thus may help the body ward off an infection by a cold or flu virus. The herb is sold in tincture, pill, and tea form. However there is a debate about its effectiveness. Most doctors do agree that if taking it makes you feel better, then you should take it.

Goldenseal contains an antibiotic substance, ***berberine*** that seems to <u>stimulate the immune system</u>. *(Berberine is from the protoberberine group of <u>isoquinoline alkaloids</u>. Plants that contain berberine are: Berberis aquifolium (Oregon grape), Berberis vulgaris (barberry), Berberis aristata (tree turmeric)], Hydrastis canadensis (goldenseal), Phellodendron amurense (huang po) and Coptis chinensis (Chinese goldthread, huang-lian), and Tinospora cordifolia, and to a smaller extent in Argemone mexicana (prickly poppy) and Eschscholzia californica (Californian poppy).*

Berberine is usually found in the roots, rhizomes, stems, and bark. As a <u>traditional medicine</u> or dietary supplement, berberine has shown some activity against fungal infections, Candida albicans, yeast, parasites, and bacterial/viral infections. Berberine seems to exert synergistic effects with fluconazole, an anti-fungal pharmaceutical, even in drug-resistant C. albicans infections.

Some research has been undertaken into possible use against MRSA infection. Remember, berberine is considered antibiotic. When applied in vitro and in combination with methoxyhydnocarpin, berberine inhibits growth of Staphylococcus aureus and Microcystis aeruginosa, a toxic cyanobacterium. Berberine is a component of some eye drop formulations. There is some evidence it is useful in the treatment of leishmaniasis. Berberine prevents and suppresses proinflammatory cytokines and increases <u>adiponectin (a weight loss hormone)</u> expression which partly explains its versatile health effects.

<u>Eucalyptus</u>: this herb is a favorite remedy of nutritionists for loosening tight coughs. They brew its leaves into a strong tea. The leaves also can be used in a steam vaporizer to relieve coughs. *Eucalyptus is found in cough drops and cough suppressants.*

Garlic: As unpleasant as it might sound and taste, garlic is most effective for a cold when eaten raw, since cooking alters some of the herb's active ingredients. *Garlic contains selenium and sulfur, which are natural immune system boosters.* It acts as an expectorant when consumed in a tea or used with warm water for gargling. Just throwing a handful of minced garlic on top of a serving of pasta is known to help treat bacterial and viral infections.

Ginger: Ginger tea is recommended for getting rid of chills, relieving sinus and chest congestion, and nausea. You can get the same benefits by grating fresh ginger into the foods you prepare. Licorice: A common component of Japanese herbal remedies, licorice extract is believed to boost immunity. It also can be used as an expectorant for upper-respiratory congestion. Peppermint: Peppermint tea taken at the first sign of a cold can alleviate symptoms of viral infection, including cough and fever.

Summary: There is no better way to bolster your immune system than by incorporating at least five servings of fruits and vegetables into your daily diet. Pick **Guavas, Melons, Pineapple, Papaya, Oranges, and Green** and **Yellow vegetables**, including **Carrots, Spinach and Winter Squash.** Spice Up your life with **Chili peppers, Hot mustard, or Horseradish,** to help clear congestion.

Zinc: -rich foods include: **Steak, pork, crab, wheat germ, brown rice and oatmeal are high in zinc.** Warm salt water gargling three times a day, with an 8-ounce glass of warm water and a few teaspoons of salt. **Tea** with a little **honey: Echinacea** and **Goldenseal** both of which contains an antibiotic substance, **berberine. Eucalyptus: Garlic: Peppermint, Ginger** and **Licorice:** all can aid in reducing and relieve the symptoms of the common cold.

Other Treatments that help alleviate symptoms include Zinc supplements, decongestants and cough medications, antihistamines, simple analgesics and antipyretics such as ibuprofen and acetaminophen/paracetamol. The misuse of Sudafed and dextromethorphan (over-the-counter sinus decongestant and cough medications) have led to its ban in a number of countries. In adults the symptoms of a runny nose can be reduced by first generation antihistamines: however, they are associated with adverse effects such as drowsiness.

Ipratropium nasal spray may reduce the symptoms of a runny nose but there is little effect on stuffiness. Second-generation antihistamines however do not appear to be effective in reducing cold symptoms unless combined to a decongestant. Increased fluid intake improves symptoms and may shorten the illness as well as the use of cool air humidifiers. One study has found chest vapor rub to be effective at providing some symptomatic relief of nocturnal cough, congestion, and sleep difficulty. Antibiotics have no effect against viral infections and thus have no effect against the viruses that cause the common cold. There are no effective antiviral treatments other than zinc supplements or nasal sprays for the common cold.

CONSTIPATION: Constipation refers to bowel movements that are infrequent or hard to pass. Constipation is not a disease but rather it is a symptom of a medical disorder.

Signs and Symptoms: Constipation is a common cause of painful defecation. Severe constipation includes obstipation (failure to pass stool or gas) and fecal impaction.

Causes: There are of two types: (1) obstructed defecation and (2) colonic slow transit (or hypo motility). About 50% of patients evaluated for constipation at tertiary referral hospitals have obstructed defecation. This type of constipation has mechanical and functional causes. Causes of colonic slow transit constipation include*diet, *hormones, *side effects of medications, and *heavy metal toxicity.

Especially in the elderly, causes include: *insufficient dietary fiber intake, *inadequate fluid intake*decreased physical activity, *side effects of medications, *hypothyroidism, and *obstruction by colorectal cancer. Constipation can be caused or exacerbated by a low fiber diet, low liquid intake, or dieting. Many medications have constipation as a side effect. Some include (but are not limited to): opioids (e.g. common pain killers), diuretics, antidepressants, antihistamines, antispasmodics, anticonvulsants (seizure medication), and aluminum antacids.

Nutritional factors: According to experts the best foods are those with the greatest amount of fiber. Several studies show that if you increase your food intake that is rich in fiber it will help eliminate your constipation. Dietary fiber seems to be the most effective way in relieving constipation problems.

Individuals who are having this condition should consider changing their dietary intake to include fiber as the most physiologic, cheapest and simplest form of treatment. However, there are some negative sides effects involved in using fiber in your diet: which are as follows: Abdominal distention, Bloating, Flatulence, Poor taste. Due to the side effects of too much fiber, individuals are advised to use **twenty five** to **thirty grams of fiber** per day.

Also, an individual needs to consume fiber at a rate of one gram per hundred calories of food consumed. Fibers are available in two types: insoluble and soluble fiber. It's important to note that soluble fiber has the ability to absorb water and produce a soft stool. On the other hand the insoluble fiber increases the bulk. These two types of fibers can be found in different types of plant foods. It is best to also drink lots of water. Fiber will work better if you drink enough fluids. Below is a list of the best foods for preventing constipation:

- Prunes – most doctors usually advise their patients to drink prune juice or eat prunes to relieve constipation. It is one of the most popular home remedies that people can easily avail. Prunes contain fiber, potassium and vitamin "A". Also, a quarter cup of prunes daily is enough to prevent constipation unless you are taking opioid type of medication.
- Flaxseed – these are tiny seeds from the flax plant. They are rich in omega 3 fatty acids, fiber, vitamins, and minerals. Ground flaxseed is best and can be put in or on cereals and salads or used in baking.
- Pears – Pears are an excellent source of vitamin C and insoluble fiber. It is a common home remedy for constipation. It mostly adds bulk to the stool.
- Apple juice is also a popular food for constipation. It contains pectin, a soluble fiber which softens and increases the bulk of the stool and helps in bowel movements.
- Banana –A ripe banana relieves constipation. It also has high content of pectin that helps in bowel movements. However, a green banana should be avoided since they can cause constipation. One ripe banana a day promotes good bowel movements.
- Whole grain – This food is rich in fiber and will speed up colonic movement and thus whole grains increase the bowel frequency and stool output. Whole wheat bread, especially stone ground whole wheat bread, is another common home remedy for preventing as well as treating constipation.

Other Recommendations: Remember fiber foods and water for preventing and treating constipation are key. Other treatments include more physical activity, changes in dietary habits, laxatives, enemas, biofeedback, and even surgery for obstructive constipation. Because **constipation is a symptom, not a disease,** effective treatment of constipation may require first determining the cause. Healthy bowels can make a big difference in your state of health.

All body cells take in nutrients to nourish themselves from the small intestine, and then these cells need to get rid of the waste material generated. The body must eliminate this waste efficiently or the toxic overload results in illness and disease and even death. Using bowel cleansers can be very helpful. Some of the most popular cleansers contain bentonite clay, psyllium husk, and herbs.

DEPRESSION: Depression is known by many different terms. For example, Major depressive disorder (also known as MDD), recurrent depressive disorder (RDD), clinical depression, major depression, unipolar depression, or unipolar disorder. Depression is a mental disorder characterized by an all-encompassing low mood and or accompanied by low self-esteem, and by loss of interest or pleasure in normally enjoyable activities. It is also characterized by a sleep disorder. **The term "depression" is ambiguous.** It is often used to denote this syndrome but may refer to other mood disorders or to lower mood states lacking clinical significance. *Major depressive disorder (MDD) is a disabling condition* that adversely affects a person's family, work or school life, sleeping and eating habits, and general health.

In the United States, around 3.4% of people with major depression commit suicide, and up to 60% of people who commit suicide had depression or another mood disorder. The diagnosis of major depressive disorder is based on the patient's self-reported experiences, behavior reported by relatives or friends, and a mental status exam.

<u>There is no laboratory test for major depression</u>, although physicians generally request tests for physical conditions that may cause similar symptoms. The most common time of onset is between the ages of 20 and 30 years, with a later peak between 30 and 40 years. Depressed individuals have shorter life expectancies than those without depression, in part because of greater susceptibility to medical illnesses and suicide. Note, many times medications affect the risk of suicide.

Signs and Symptoms: A person having a major depressive episode usually exhibits a very low mood, which pervades all aspects of life, and an inability to experience pleasure in activities that were formerly enjoyed. Depressed people may be preoccupied with, or ruminate over, thoughts and feelings of worthlessness, inappropriate guilt or regret, helplessness, hopelessness, and self-hatred. In severe cases, depressed people may have symptoms of psychosis. These symptoms include delusions or, less commonly, hallucinations, usually unpleasant.

Other symptoms of depression include poor concentration and memory (especially in those with melancholic or psychotic features), withdrawal from social situations and activities, reduced sex drive, and thoughts of death or suicide. Insomnia is common among the depressed. Typically, a person wakes very early and cannot get back to sleep. Insomnia affects at least 80% of depressed people.

Over-sleeping or hypersomnia can also happen. Some antidepressants may also cause insomnia due to their stimulating effect. A depressed person may report multiple physical symptoms such as fatigue, headaches, or digestive problems. Physical complaints seem to be the most common presenting problem in developing countries. Appetite often decreases, with resulting weight loss, although increased appetite and weight gain occasionally occur. Family and friends may notice that the person's behavior is either agitated or lethargic.

Older depressed people may have cognitive symptoms of recent onset, such as forgetfulness, and a more noticeable slowing of movements. Depression often coexists with physical disorders common among the elderly, such as stroke, other cardiovascular diseases, Parkinson's disease, and chronic obstructive pulmonary disease.

Depressed children may often display an irritable mood rather than a depressed mood, and show varying symptoms depending on age and situation. Most lose interest in school and show a decline in academic performance. They may be described as clingy, demanding, dependent, or insecure. Diagnosis may be delayed or missed when symptoms are interpreted as normal moodiness. Depression often coexists with attention-deficit hyperactivity disorder (ADHD), complicating the diagnosis and treatment of both.

Causes: Proposed causes include psychological, psycho-social, trauma, hereditary, evolutionary and biological factors and loss of a family member, friend or loss of a job. Certain types of long-term drug use as well as poor nutrition can cause and/or worsen depressive symptoms.

Nutritional factors: In many cases, certain foods have been proven to be more effective than prescribed antidepressants. Some of these foods include:

Salmon: Fish are high in healthy omega-3 fatty acids, and salmon has some of the highest levels of these fats. Omega-3 fatty acids help keep cells pliable and strong, and they greatly help to treat depression. They are also high in tryptophan, an amino acid used to make natural antidepressant hormones such as serotonin.

Spinach: B vitamins, especially vitamin B9, have been known to play a role in treating depression in some people. Spinach has a high concentration of folate, (vitamin B9), that plays a significantly important role in treating depression.

Oats and oatmeal have high levels of tryptophan. This is an amino acid used by the brain to make serotonin, which is something many anti-depressant drugs try to create.

Quinoa is a seed that is believed to have the highest level of protein in the vegetable kingdom. It also has sugars that are released slowly, which limits the highs and lows of regular sugar intake, which can affect depression.

Broccoli helps to stabilize blood sugar levels. Our moods are affected by the level of blood sugar, and that can affect depression.

Cheeses contain a significant amount of tyrosine, an amino acid used by the brain to make dopamine, a neuro-transmitter that acts as a natural antidepressant.

Turkey, chicken and duck (dark meat): contain significant levels of tyrosine, an amino-acid used by the brain to produce dopamine and norepinephrine, natural chemicals known to reduce the risk of depression.

Other Recommendations: Physical exercise and a healthy diet consisting of 30% complex carbohydrates, 30% proteins, 30% healthy fats is recommended for management of all degrees of depression, but absolutely no artificial non-nutritive sweetener, and high fructose corn syrup and no trans-fats such as margarine, shortening or other products that contain hydrogenated oils.

Note: only omega 3 and 6 fatty acids, canola oil and or olive oil or coconut oil should be consumed. There are three other common medical treatments for depression. They are medication, psychotherapy, and electroconvulsive therapy. Psychotherapy is the treatment of choice for people under 18, while electroconvulsive therapy is used only as a last resort.

Care is usually given on an outpatient basis, whereas treatment in an inpatient unit is considered if there is a significant risk to self or others. Treatment options are much more limited in developing countries, where access to mental health staff, medication, and psychotherapy is often difficult.

Development of mental health services is minimal in many countries, especially where depression is viewed as a phenomenon of the developed world despite evidence to the contrary, and not as an inherently life-threatening condition. Other treatments are based on theories of personality, interpersonal communication, and learning.

Most biological theories focus on the monoamine chemicals: serotonin, norepinephrine and dopamine, which are made naturally from certain amino acids (tyrosine and tryptophan) found in proteins and are present in the brain to assist communication between nerve cells. Typically, patients are treated with antidepressant medication rather than food nutrients (natural foods high in certain amino-acids). In some cases, they also receive psychotherapy or counseling.

DEMENTIA: (See also **ALZHEIMER**) Dementia **is** a metabolic age-related degenerative brain disorder.

Signs and Symptoms: Dementia manifests as a progressive deterioration of memory, cognitive and mental functioning and the inability to carry out activities of daily living.

Causes: (1)*a reduced level of acetylcholine*, (a key neurotransmitter in the brain that is especially important for memory): (2) the formation of neurofibrillary tangles and plaques (scars) composed of various protein and cellular debris or toxins. The result of these toxins or debris is loss of brain cells. AD is a chronic degenerative disease in which both genetic factors and environmental factors play a role. For example, *oxidative damage, *traumatic brain injury, *chronic exposure to aluminum and or silicon (from antacids, antiperspirants, aluminum pots and pans) and *exposure to toxins (chemicals and frying foods in burnt oils) from environmental sources: all of which produce scar tissue in the brain, have all been implicated as causative factors.

Nutritional factors: A lack of folic acid, vitamin B12 and a lack of omega-3 fatty acids (especially DHA from fish oils) play major roles in the development and/or progression of AD (Dementia). Also, a lack of antioxidants causes AD due to free radicals and oxidative damage. Some examples of nutrients that can be used to prevent or treat AD are: antioxidants such as carotenes, vitamins C and E, and anti-inflammatory nutrients such as flavonoid-rich fruits. (See pg 142).

 Ones diet should **contain lots** of (1) flavonoid-rich fruits (especially citrus and berries) and (2) carotene-rich vegetables, such as carrots, yams, and squash, whole grain carbohydrates and (3) omega-3 rich cold water fish or fish oil and (4) folic acid and vitamin B12 foods such a dark leafy green vegetables and/or Brewer's yeast. This diet should **limit** (1) sweets (especially high fructose corn syrup and artificial, nonnutritive sweeteners), (2) trans fats like margarine and shortening, and (3) any highly processed foods but especially those containing non-nutritive (artificial) sweeteners and those containing hydrogenated oils (even ice cream, peanut butter, mayonnaise or miracle whip **if they contain hydrogenated oils**). The risk of getting AD would be reduced if we made everything from scratch (i.e., without preservatives and highly processed ingredients). Note: even lard (a saturated fat) is better than shortening (a transfat). Elderly people's mental function is directly related to their nutritional status. It is noteworthy that: (1) **ginkgo**

biloba extract, (2) **acetyl –L carnitine** (*the amino acid that "transports long-chain fatty acids* and (3) **turmeric**, the spice that contains curcumin: are currently being investigated for their effects in the prevention of AD.

DIABETES MELLITUS: Diabetes mellitus, or simply "diabetes", is more of a group of metabolic disorders involving insulin in which a person has high blood sugar: either because (1) the body does not produce enough insulin, or (2) because damaged receptors on cell membranes are resistant to insulin. The latter is known as "insulin resistance".

There are basically two types of diabetes. Type 1 diabetes mellitus is characterized by loss of the insulin-producing beta cells of the Islets of Langerhans in the pancreas, leading to no insulin being produced. This type can be further classified as immune-mediated or idiopathic. The majority of type 1 diabetes is of the immune-mediated nature, in which beta cell loss is a T-cell-mediated autoimmune attack that, in some individuals, is triggered by an infection.

 There is no known preventive measure against type 1 diabetes except, maybe, eating foods high in anti-oxidants and anti-inflammatory nutrients (natural fruits and vegetables, especially sweet potatoes blue-berries kidney beans, onions, etc.) and totally eliminating sugar, artificial sweeteners and trans-fats (hydrogenated oils) and foods sprayed with toxic chemicals.

Receptor sensitivity and responsiveness to insulin are usually normal, especially in the early stages. Type 2 diabetes mellitus is the common type and is characterized by insulin resistance, and maybe combined with a reduction in insulin secretion. The defective responsiveness of body tissues to insulin is believed to involve the damaged insulin receptor.

In the early stage of type 2 diabetes, the predominant abnormality is reduced insulin sensitivity due to damaged insulin receptors. Reduced insulin sensitivity and/or the damaged insulin receptor is also referred to as insulin resistance. At an early stage, reduced glucose production by the liver can be reversed by a variety of measures, i.e. low carbohydrate diet with appropriate amounts of vegetables and fruit (anti-oxidants and anti-inflammatory nutrients) and medications that improve insulin sensitivity, i.e., Glucophage (Metformin). [*However, Glucophage usually causes weight gain, as well as an increase in blood levels of triglycerides and cholesterol. This is because Glucophage/Metformin interferes with or blocks gluconeogenesis, the fat burning process located in the liver*].

Signs and Symptoms: The classical symptoms of untreated diabetes are: weight loss, polyuria (frequent urination), polydipsia (increased thirst) and polyphagia (increased hunger). Symptoms may develop rapidly (weeks or months) in type 1 diabetes, while they usually develop much more slowly and subtly in type 2 diabetes.

Prolonged high blood glucose can cause glucose absorption in the lens of the eye, which leads to changes in its shape, resulting in vision changes. Blurred vision is a common complaint leading to a diabetes diagnosis. Type 1 diabetes should always be suspected in cases of rapid vision change, whereas with type 2 diabetes, change is generally more gradual, but should still be suspected. A number of skin rashes that can occur in diabetes are collectively known as diabetic dermatomes.

Diabetic emergencies: people (usually with type 1 diabetes) may present with diabetic ketoacidosis, a state of metabolic deregulation characterized by the smell of acetone, a rapid, deep breathing known as Kussmaul breathing, nausea, vomiting and abdominal pain, and altered states of consciousness. A rare but equally severe possibility is hyperosmolar non-ketotic state, which is more common in type 2 diabetes and is mainly the result of dehydration.

Causes of Type 1 Diabetes. In type 1 diabetes, the body no longer makes insulin because the body's own immune system attacked and destroyed the <u>pancreatic</u> <u>beta cells</u> where insulin is made. The cause of this isn't entirely clear but it may include genetic risk factors and environmental factors. One theory is that type 1 diabetes may occur after having a specific viral infection. People with type 1 diabetes must take insulin every day in order to live. There is no known way to prevent or cure type 1 diabetes, but it can be controlled by eating low glycemic foods that keep blood glucose levels low, <110mg/dl.

Causes of Type 2 Diabetes. Type 2 diabetes is the most common form of diabetes. In type 2 diabetes, the body either doesn't make enough insulin or can't use its own insulin as well as it should. The risk of having type 2 diabetes increases as a person gets older. The cause of type 2 diabetes is largely unknown, but genetics, diet and lifestyle clearly play a role. Type 2 diabetes has been linked to obesity, genetic risk factors, and inactivity. Some racial and ethnic groups are at higher risk for type 2 diabetes. These include American Indians, African Americans, Hispanics/Latinos, Asian Americans and Pacific Islanders. There is no known cure for type 2 diabetes until someone figures out how to correct or heal the damaged insulin receptors, but it can be controlled in the same manner as type 1 diabetes.

Nutritional factors: People suffering from diabetes need to eat healthy in order to keep their blood sugar levels under control. Though they are not left with much variety, as far as carbohydrates are concerned: <u>vegetables are unlimited</u>. The kidney <u>bean</u> and <u>sweet potato</u> are good options. If cooked with care, they both taste awesome and no less than a delicacy. Both have great fiber content and are rich in low glycemic carbohydrates.

Also, beans and sweet potatoes are rich in soluble fiber which effectively reduces the blood sugar levels. Lettuce and tomatoes are also good vegetables for diabetics. People who wish to cut down on their weight can have plenty of lettuce as well as tomatoes as they have low carbohydrate content and also control levels of blood sugar.

Onion, be it raw or cooked, is also an effective home remedy. It effectively reduces blood sugar levels on its own. Onions contain anti-diabetic compounds - namely allyl propyl disulphide and allicin. These medicinal nutrients help the pancreas synthesize insulin and its release. These nutrients may even heal the damaged insulin receptors.

A balanced diet, well supplemented with vegetables, fruit and diluted unsweetened juices (tomato juice is great) should be ideally eaten daily. All individuals, but especially those with diabetes, need to cut down on the intake of sweets and unhealthy fats that are contained in most processed foods: especially those processed foods made with artificial nonnutritive sweeteners and/or hydrogenated oils such as lunch meat. Hydrogenated oils are another name for "trans-fats". Besides eating nutritiously, physical exercise can control blood sugar.

GLUCONEOGENESIS (THE FAT-BURNING PROCESS IN THE LIVER)

The production of glucose from triglycerides (body fats) is called gluconeogenesis and it occurs in the liver. Gluconeogenesis is known as the fat burning process.

When the blood sugar (**glucose**) level is low, then the pancreas doesn't release any **Insulin**. Therefore the Insulin level in the blood stream is low. Whenever both the glucose level and the Insulin level in the blood stream are low, then the pancreas releases **Glucagon** the good (healing)

93

hormone. Glucagon then goes to the fat cell and triggers the release of triglycerides (body fat) into the blood stream and then initiates the transport of this fat molecule to the liver where these fat molecules (triglycerides) are converted to glucose. **This chemical process is called gluconeogenesis.**

(NOTE: Glucagon is considered the fat burning hormone. And Insulin is considered the fat storing hormone).

The Fat burning furnace is a term I coined to illustrate the **gluconeogensis process in the liver** where body fat (triglyceride) molecules are converted (oxidized or changed) to glucose. The diabetic medicine Metformin (Glucophage) actually blocks gluconeogenesis. Metformin (Glucophage) blocks or *gums-up* an enzyme process necessary for the fat burning process to change body fat into glucose. In this way Metformin (Glucophage) does lowers the glucose level in the blood stream but at the expense of raising triglyceride and cholesterol levels and causing many more medical problems.

DIARRHEA: Diarrhea is defined by the World Health Organization (WHO) as having three or more loose or liquid stools per day, or as having more stools than is normal for that person. It is not really a disease but rather a symptom associated with many causes or diseases. The loss of fluids through diarrhea can cause dehydration and electrolyte disturbances such as potassium deficiency or other salt imbalances. It is the second most common cause of infant deaths worldwide.

Signs, Symptoms and Causes:

Secretory diarrhea means that there is an increase in the active secretion, or there is an inhibition of absorption of fluids. There is little to no structural damage. The most common cause of this type

94

of diarrhea is a *cholera toxin* that stimulates the secretion of anions, especially chloride ions. Therefore, to maintain a charge balance in the lumen, sodium is carried with it, along with water. In this type of diarrhea intestinal fluid secretion is isotonic with plasma. *It continues even when there is no oral food intake.*

Osmotic diarrhea occurs when too much water is drawn into the bowels. If a person drinks solutions with excessive sugar or excessive salt, these can draw water from the blood stream into the bowel and cause osmotic diarrhea. Osmotic diarrhea can also be the result of pancreatic disease or *Celiac disease*, in which the nutrients are left in the lumen to pull in water.

Or it can be caused by osmotic laxatives (which work to alleviate constipation by drawing water into the bowels). In healthy individuals, too much magnesium or vitamin C or undigested lactose can produce osmotic diarrhea and distention of the bowel. A person who has lactose intolerance can have difficulty absorbing lactose after an extraordinarily high intake of dairy products. Excess fructose intake can also cause diarrhea in persons who have fructose malabsorption. Fruits with high-fructose content are more absorbable and less likely to cause diarrhea. Sugar alcohols, such as sorbitol (often found in sugar-free foods), are difficult for the body to absorb and, in large amounts, may lead to osmotic diarrhea. In most of these cases, osmotic diarrhea stops when offending agent (e.g. milk, sorbitol, etc.) is stopped.

Exudative diarrhea occurs with the presence of blood and pus in the stool. This occurs with *inflammatory bowel diseases*, such as Crohn's disease or ulcerative colitis, and other severe infections such as *E. coli or other forms of food poisoning*.

Motility-related diarrhea is caused by the rapid movement of food through the intestines (hypermotility). If the food moves too quickly through the gastrointestinal tract, there is not enough time for sufficient nutrients and water to be absorbed. This can be due to a vagotomy, a form of stomach surgery or diabetic neuropathy. Hyperthyroidism can produce hypermotility and lead to diarrhea. Hypermotility can be observed in people who have had portions of their bowel removed, allowing less total time for absorption of nutrients.

Inflammatory diarrhea occurs when there is damage to the mucosal lining or brush border, which leads to a passive loss of protein-rich fluids, and a decreased ability to absorb these lost fluids. It can be caused by bacterial infections, viral infections, parasitic infections, or autoimmune problems such as inflammatory bowel diseases, IBD. It can also be caused by tuberculosis, colon cancer, and enteritis.

Dysentery is not diarrhea: it is a symptom. Loose frequent stools with visible blood is called Dysentery. The blood is a sign of an invasion of bowel tissue. *Dysentery is a symptom of, among others, Shigella, Entamoeba histolytica, and Salmonella infections.* Diarrhea in children is most commonly due to viral gastroenteritis with rotavirus. In travelers, however, bacterial infections predominate. Various toxins in mushroom and drugs can also cause acute diarrhea.

Chronic diarrhea can be the part of the presentations of a number of chronic medical conditions affecting the intestine. Common causes include ulcerative colitis, Crohn's disease, microscopic colitis, celiac disease, irritable bowel syndrome and bile acid malabsorption.

Infectious diarrhea: There are many causes of infectious diarrhea, which include viruses, bacteria and parasites. Norovirus is the most common cause of viral diarrhea in adults, but rotavirus is the most common cause in children under five years old. Adenovirus and astroviruses cause a significant number of infections.

The bacterium Campylobacter is a common cause of bacterial diarrhea, but infections by Salmonellae, Shigellae and some strains of Escherichia coli (E.coli) are more frequent. In the elderly, particularly those who have been treated with antibiotics for unrelated infections, a toxin produced by Clostridium difficile often causes severe diarrhea.

Parasites do not often cause diarrhea except for the protozoan Giardia, which can cause chronic infections if these are not diagnosed and treated with drugs such as metronidazole. Other infectious agents such as parasites and bacterial toxins also occur. In sanitary living conditions where there is ample food and a supply of clean water, an otherwise healthy person usually recovers from viral infections in a few days. However, for ill or malnourished individuals, diarrhea can lead to severe dehydration and can become life-threatening.

Enzyme deficiencies or mucosal abnormality can cause diarrhea, as in food allergy and food intolerance, e.g. celiac disease (gluten intolerance), lactose intolerance (intolerance to milk sugar), and fructose malabsorption: pernicious anemia, or impaired bowel function due to the inability to absorb vitamin B12, loss of pancreatic secretions, which may be due to cystic fibrosis or pancreatitis, structural defects, like short bowel syndrome (surgically removed bowel) and radiation fibrosis, such as usually follows cancer treatment and other drugs, including agents used in chemotherapy: and certain diet drugs, like orlistat, which inhibits the absorption of fat. Ulcerative colitis is marked by chronic bloody diarrhea and inflammation and mostly affects the distal colon near the rectum.

Another possible cause of diarrhea is irritable bowel syndrome (IBS) which usually presents with abdominal discomfort relieved by defecation and unusual stool (diarrhea or constipation) for at least 3 days a week over the previous 3 months. Symptoms of diarrhea-predominant IBS can be managed through a combination of dietary changes, soluble fiber supplements, and/or medications such as loperamide or codeine.

About 30% of patients with diarrhea-predominant IBS (Irritable bowel syndrome) have bile acid malabsorption.

Other causes of diarrhea: diarrhea can be caused by ischemic bowel disease. This usually affects older people and can be due to blocked arteries. Microscopic colitis, a type of inflammatory bowel disease where changes are only seen on histological examination of colonic biopsies. Bile salt malabsorption (primary bile acid diarrhea) where excessive bile acids in the colon produce a secretory diarrhea. Some hormones (e.g., serotonin) can cause diarrhea if excreted in excess (usually from a hormone secreting tumor). Chronic mild diarrhea in infants and toddlers may occur with no obvious cause and with no other ill effects: this condition is called toddler's diarrhea.

Nutritional factors: Oral rehydration solutions containing modest amounts of salt and zinc are the treatment of choice. Vomiting often occurs during the first hour, but this seldom prevents successful rehydration as most of the fluid is still absorbed. Homemade solutions include (isotonic) salted drinks (e.g. salted rice water or a salted yogurt drink) and vegetable or chicken soup with salt.

If available, bananas or supplemental potassium, as well as supplemental zinc, can be added to or given with this homemade solution. It's also recommended that persons with diarrhea, if able, continue or resume eating as this speeds recovery of normal intestinal function and generally leads to diarrhea of shorter duration. Plain non-flavored water as well as chicken broth and vegetable soups should be first on the list to treat diarrhea. There are commercial solutions such as Pedialyte, and relief agencies such as UNICEF widely distribute packets of salts and real sugar.

A homemade solution can be made by adding between one-half to one teaspoon of salt (about 2-3 grams) and six teaspoons sugar (about 18 grams) to one liter of water. A homemade oral rehydration solution (ORS) should have the "taste of tears."

Also **green bananas, cheese, zinc, chicken noodle soup** and **isotonic water** may be useful to correct most diarrheas. Diarrhea can be treated with anti-motility agents (such as loperamide / Lomotil, donnatal, etc.).

EAR INFECTION (OTITIS MEDIA): Otitis media (Latin) is a middle ear infection due to inflammation of the middle ear. It occurs in the area between the tympanic membrane and the inner ear, including a duct known as the Eustachian Tube, (a duct that connects the oral cavity with the middle ear. Inflammation and infection is one of the most common causes of an earache (pain). Other causes of ear ache include: otitis externa (infection of the outer ear canal): allergies (most of such allergies come from food, and toxic inhalations): and diseases such as cancers of any structure that shares the same nerve supply with the ear. However, painful, otitis media is not life threatening and usually heals on its own within 2–6 weeks. Acute ear infections (aka, Acute Otitis Media) can be caused by an upper respiratory infection, (i.e. common cold caused by a viral infection), that spreads to the ears.

Signs and Symptoms of an ear infection include: earache, fullness and pressure or pain in the ear, and a fever as high as 103°F, or even higher. Children may pull their ears to relieve the pressure. They may be irritable or restless, have a nasal discharge, diminished

CARLA D. O. SHARBONO, M.D.

appetite, or cry at night when lying down. If symptoms become severe or are untreated, there is danger of potential hearing loss, which may lead to impairment of language skills or intellectual development.

If untreated AOM can also lead to hearing loss, perforation of the eardrum, and even more serious medical conditions. In adults, symptoms often include nasal congestion, nausea and diarrhea, earache, chills, fever, and muffled hearing. When the middle ear becomes suddenly or acutely infected, pressure builds up behind the eardrum (tympanic membrane), frequently causing intense pain. It may result in bullous myringitis (myring means "eardrum"), which means that the tympanic membrane is blistered and inflamed.

In severe or untreated cases, the tympanic membrane may rupture, allowing the pus in the middle ear space to drain into the outer ear canal. If there is enough fluid, i.e. "pus", this drainage may be obvious. In a simple case of acute otitis media in an otherwise healthy person, the body's defenses are likely to resolve the infection and the ear drum nearly always heals. However, if the infection and eardrum perforation does not resolve, drainage from the middle ear can become a chronic condition.

Note: as long as there is active middle ear infection, the eardrum will not heal.

Chronic suppurative otitis media is a stage of ear disease in which there is chronic infection of the middle ear, a perforated eardrum and discharge, for at least two weeks. Serous otitis media, is the term that denotes a simple fluid collection within the middle ear behind an intact eardrum.

Causes: Otitis media is most commonly caused by an infection within the middle ear due to viral, bacterial, or fungal pathogens. The most common bacterial pathogen is Streptococcus pneumoniae. Others include Pseudomonas aeruginosa, non-typeable Haemophilus influenzae, and Moraxella catarrhalis. Among older adolescents and young adults, the most common cause of ear infections is Haemophilus influenzae.

Viruses such as respiratory syncytial virus (RSV) and those viruses that cause the common cold may also result in otitis media by damaging the normal defenses of the epithelial cells in the upper respiratory tract. A major risk factor or cause for developing otitis media is Eustachian tube dysfunction, which leads to the ineffective clearing of bacteria from the middle ear. Inflammation and mucus from the infection causes the Eustachian tube to swell shut, trapping bacteria in the middle ear cavity.

(The function of the Eustachian tube is to provide an outlet for mucus and equalize pressure changes between the middle ear and the oral cavity. Normally closed, it opens to allow drainage of secretions into the throat. If this does not occur properly, an air pocket forms and the negative pressure sweeps the bacteria and/or virus into the middle ear. When this occurs, germs have a perfect environment to flourish).

Specialized cells in the middle ear manufacture fluid that helps keep out invading germs. If the Eustachian tube becomes so swollen that the fluid becomes trapped in the middle ear, the area can become inflamed and an infection sets in. Note: If the infection is bacterial, symptoms may clear up with antibiotics, but the cough and runny nose may not get better, due to the virus.

Chronically enlarged adenoids (lymph tissue that grows in the nose) may also cause blockage of the Eustachian tubes, leading to congestion and fluid in the middle ear. Although enlarged adenoids are the obvious cause of Eustachian tube blockage and the resulting ear congestion, they point to a deeper disorder. Adenoids do not enlarge without a cause: so cures should focus on correcting conditions that led to adenoid enlargement.

The Acid / Alkaline Balance. Probably the most important thing we can do with our diet for health and vitality is to maintain a proper acid-alkaline balance. In healthy people, a proper balance is normally maintained through a buffering system. This balance depends on a healthy digestive system as well as a healthy liver. Poor assimilation and elimination, lack of digestive enzymes, severe infections or illness, second-hand smoke or drug use all interfere with this buffering system.

Acidic wastes are the end products of cellular metabolism and must not be allowed to build up, so the body goes to great lengths to neutralize and detoxify these acids. A diet balanced in acid-alkaline foods, usually found in vegetables, is essential for the body to meet this goal.

 If the body cannot detoxify, it puts excessive demands on the immune system. "Detox" is essential in reducing the risk of the over production of mucus, a leading cause of ear infections. While bacteria can be the direct cause of an ear infection, other culprits are usually the result of an "insult" to the body, such as an allergic reaction or a weakened immune system, imbalances in the digestive system, or inflammation of the mucous membranes (leading to excess mucus secretion).

When bacteria find their way into the warm, moist environment of the middle ear, they can create major problems, turning inflammation into infection and provoking fever and pain as well as other symptoms. A compromised (poor) Immune System, can be a very significant cause of recurring ear infections, especially in young children, who are often linked to a poor immune system and weakened resistance due to inadequate nutrition, food allergies, environmental toxins and emotional stress.

Too often, parents and doctors treat the symptoms of ear infections with antibiotics without looking for the cause of the problem.

Antibiotics may work initially, but don't solve the ongoing problem of recurrent ear infections. While antibiotics do kill harmful bacteria, they also indiscriminately destroy beneficial intestinal bacteria. This upsets the delicate balance needed for good digestion and elimination, priming the internal environment for pathogen organisms such as harmful bacteria and Candida Albicans (an overgrowth of a naturally occurring yeast).

Unchecked, these organisms can cause further problems and create a vicious cycle of more ear infections, more antibiotics and more imbalance. With each "incident," the immune system becomes weaker, making each successive illness harder to fight off. Overuse of antibiotics—the quick-fix solution—thus contributes to long-term health problems.

A better solution is to strengthen the immune system with foods high in anti-oxidants (vegetables and fruit). See pg 182. Damage caused by overuse of antibiotics can be mitigated by preparations called "probiotics." Low humidity may be a contributing factor in chronic ear infections.

A possible explanation is that low humidity may induce nasal swelling and reduce drainage of the Eustachian tube, or it may dry the hairs out in the Eustachian tube, leading to dysfunction and resulting in increased mucus.

Note: Bottle fed babies are often left lying down in a crib or on their backs. Feeding an infant on its back can lead to regurgitation into the middle ear. If the head is resting too low, the milk can back up into the ears and provide a breeding ground for bacteria, causing infection.

Allergies to foods, pollen, dust, mold, animal dander, smoke, fumes, or other environmental toxins can also cause otitis media symptoms, because anything that irritates or inflames the mucous membranes will stimulate excess mucus secretion.

 Diet, allergies and stress are the most likely sources of earaches when a fever is not involved. If you eat too many sweets or fried foods as well as processed foods containing trans-fats, the immune system (which is regulated in part by a fatty acid balance) may mistakenly launch an attack on the body, resulting in inflammation.

Additionally, the structure and metabolism of nerve cells, their energy supply and functional integrity are all related to the constant availability of nutrients. Stress, coffee, tea, and colas drain potassium and disrupt inner ear fluid balance. Having the right balance of sodium and potassium is extremely important, because inner ear fluids feed a large portion of the sensory cells in the ears.

 A Magnesium Deficiency also plays a significant role in the proper function of the inner ear. Magnesium is important to enzymatic function and circulatory health. Second-hand smoke can push children with ear problems toward infections by creating pollutant-filled air that can lead to Eustachian tube congestion. Soot and smoke from a wood-burning stove can also load the air with toxins.

Being exposed to smoke can reduce the oxygen carrying capacity of the blood by nearly one-third. Ear infections also occur after exposure to cold wind or water, although infections can appear at any time. High altitudes and cold climates increase the risk of these infections. Decompression during air travel can also be a trigger.

An imbalance in the digestive system is a common cause of excess mucous. When digestive organs become irritated or inflamed, excess mucous develops nearly everywhere in the body. This is often followed by headaches, postnasal drip, sinus inflammation, digestive disorders, recurrent colds and ear infections.

Dairy products increase mucus production, and may be an underlying cause of ear infections. If excess mucus did not exist in the first place, the Eustachian would not become so congested, and germs would not have such a good place to thrive. Further, many children are lactose deficient. This means that they do not have the ability to make enough of the digestive enzyme "lactase" to digest lactose, a component of milk. This can cause a host of digestive symptoms including diarrhea, bloating, gas, and stomachaches.

Sugar, found in most packaged or processed foods and soda in one form or another, is especially good at producing excessive mucus in the body. Salt is another major cause of too much mucus. There are other causes, but most frequently it is an unbalanced diet. Most people think of excess mucus in terms of runny noses and sinusitis. These are certainly common complaints, but not the only place in the body where excess mucus may be a problem. It is important to know that mucus is a natural and normal secretion of the body. In the usual small amounts, it lubricates and protects the delicate mucous membranes found throughout the body.

It is when mucus accumulates or is produced in excess amounts that it interferes with the normal action of the affected tissues or organs. Excess nasal mucus may not only compromise the ears, but also the stomach, intestinal tract, fallopian tubes, ducts, or any other mucous membrane-lined part of the body. Bacterial infection, if present, is the result of internal congestion or inflammation caused excess mucous. This condition can be relieved only when the cause of the body's excess mucus production is corrected.

Too Many Carbohydrates is definitely a major cause of otitis media. Any carbohydrate—even the best, unrefined whole wheat bread—

if consumed in excess, can create an increase in mucus production. The most frequent dietary problem is an extremely unbalanced diet, with excessive consumption of carbohydrates. This situation is worse if refined carbohydrates such as devitalized white bread, white rice, or sugar are eaten regularly, causing excess acid and mucus to build up in body tissues. Infants and children who eat mostly refined starches often exhibit this condition of runny nose congestion and earache.

Food Allergies cause Excess Mucus. Any food allergy or sensitivity can cause excess mucus production. Since food allergies and sensitivities are one of the major causes of recurrent ear infections in children, it is wise to first eliminate the foods most frequently associated with excess mucus production: wheat, dairy products, sugar, and eggs. Also exclude all refined carbohydrates, sugar, salt, pepper, sodas, strong spices and junk foods.

Coffee or tea (except herbal without caffeine) should be removed as well. Removing sugar and sugar-laden juices such as soda pop and even many juices will eliminate 50-70% of the remaining ear infections. Be patient. It can take a full month to eliminate all the excess mucus from the body that is caused by eating the wrong foods, but it can significantly reduce the symptoms.

Why Proper Bowel Function is Important! If the inflammation reaches the point where toxins seep through the irritated and sometimes thinned lining of the gut, the stage is set for the creation of disease anywhere in the body. If the organs of elimination are not working effectively, or are overburdened by this toxic/irritant excess, an excess mucus condition will develop. That is why it is so important to establish and maintain proper bowel function.

For hundreds of years, the large intestine has been thought to play a major role in a wide range of diseases. Treatment should address changing the intestinal micro flora, increasing peristaltic activity, and overcoming stasis without resorting to toxic measures. This can be done with diet, exercise, herbal and homeopathic medications, enemas and other natural and non-invasive methods, such as <u>cascara and senna</u>. It is also important to drink adequate pure water and avoid excess salt and sugar.

Nutritional factors. Consuming flax seed oil, olive oil, crushed walnut and pumpkin seeds will improve otitis media. <u>Flaxseed oil, olive oil, walnut or pumpkin oils vegetable and fruit should be used first as these reduce inflammation as well as reduce the secretion of excess mucous.</u> Citrus juices such as grapefruit and lemon, if not too concentrated, can help to break up congestion and cure ear infections.

Fresh apple juice seems to be easier on the stomach. Onions and odorless garlic capsules are very useful mucus solvents, as well as all berries (strawberries, blackberries, raspberries, cranberries, etc.) **Pineapple**, if not excessively sweet, <u>is a good mucus solvent</u>, as are whole <u>oranges, grapefruits, lemons, cherries, and tomatoes.</u>

<u>Fresh squeezed **vegetable juices** not only help the body eliminate mucus, but nourish and rebuild tissues and help neutralize acidic waste.</u> Some of the tastiest vegetables juices are combinations of several different vegetables, such as carrot, beet, and ginger. Try the ones that are low in added sugar. **Zinc** supplementation have been shown to relieve symptoms when severe malnutrition causes ear ache. **Omega-3 fatty acids** (found in fatty fish and flax oil) may also reduce the risk of an ear infection.

Other Dietary Recommendations. Many people with ear infections need to avoid dairy products and wheat for at least 2 months, if not permanently, as well as the other foods mentioned earlier. Minimize the consumption of cow's milk, and highly processed meat products and carbohydrates (sweets).

After eliminating mucus-forming foods for at least a month it is time to expand the diet with the first introduced grains being brown rice and millet. If dairy products are to be given, start with goat's yogurt because it seems to cause less mucus production then cow's milk. Whole wheat in small amounts may then be added, but yeast-free if possible.

Since so many children seem to have issues with wheat, it might be better to use other grains such as rye, spelt, corn, rice or oats. Children who are breast-fed are less susceptible to ear infections. This is due in part to the immune building properties of colostrum found in the mother's milk.

A child's Eustachian tube is not positioned at the same angle as an adult's (it is shorter and lies in a more horizontal position), making children more prone to infection.

A diet balanced in acid-alkaline foods is essential for the body to meet this goal. If the body cannot naturally detoxify, it puts excessive demands on the immune system. This increases the risk of immune problems and results in the over production of mucus, a leading cause of ear infections.

Once a food is digested, it is known as "ash." Generally, meat, sugar, and grains yield an **acid ash,** whereas fruits and vegetables, especially green leafy vegetables, yield an **alkaline ash**, and fats yield a **neutral ash**. Ideally, the body maintains a neutral or slightly alkaline state (pH 7).

When a body gets too acidic (pH 4-6) one of the things that happens is the increase of mucus. As a rule, the body needs more alkaline food than acidic food. This is necessary for the pancreas to produce enzymes and for the liver to function best. **Acid foods** include meat and carbohydrate-rich foods, while **alkaline foods** are mostly fruits, vegetables, herbs, and spices. It is important not to consume excess meat protein without balancing it with enough alkaline foods of fruits and vegetables.

__The ideal ratio is 75 percent alkaline foods to 25 percent acid foods at each meal.__

Some of the most <u>alkaline foods</u> are: molasses, beans, raisins, beet greens, spinach, brewer's yeast, almonds, soybeans, celery, and most vegetables and sprouted seeds and sprouted grains. Some of <u>the most acidic foods are wheat germ, animal products, and all sugars. Others are coca-cola, catsup, cocoa, flour products, and mustard. Dairy products are fairly acidic. These include all cheeses, ice cream, custards, and milk. Prunes and plums are fruits that are also acid forming. Just because fruits have an acidic taste does not mean that it breaks down in the body to an acidic state. Most drugs and coffee cause acidic ash.</u>

Additional recommendation. <u>Be careful blowing the nose due</u> to imbalanced pressure in the Eustachian tube during an ear infection. Keep the ear canal dry. Put cotton in the ear canal when showering or bathing. Do not swim or go out in the rain during an infection.

Use hydrotherapy: soak neck bandages in cool water and apply to the inflamed ear. At the same time, put the feet in a <u>hot footbath with a tablespoon of mustard or cayenne powder</u>. Hydrotherapy can reduce the pain and swelling by drawing the blood away from the upper body.

<u>Do not become chilled: wrap the body in a blanket</u>. Place a hot water bottle, wrapped in a towel, on the aching ear. Applications of <u>compresses soaked in hot water</u> alternated with cold compresses may relieve pain and can stimulate circulation to the area to help fight infections. **Alternating hot and cold packs** may also help relieve pain. Some earaches respond better to hot treatments and others to cold treatments.

Drink lots of pure spring or filtered water: it helps to reduce mucus and eliminate toxins from the body. In cold, damp weather, **keep the feet warm** and **avoid drafts** especially near the head. Protect the neck by wearing a scarf or other covering. Vitamin and mineral deficiencies affect the immune system.

Gargling with salt water can help to clear the Eustachian tubes. Holding the head erect may help drain excess fluid from the middle ear. __Vitamin C__ helps to support the immune system and fight ear infections. Add 1 teaspoon vitamin C crystals or powder to 6 ounces of water. Take 1/2 to 1 ounce of this mixture every 1-3 hours. Reduce the dosage if it causes a stomachache or loose stools. Zinc can be very helpful when fighting acute ear infections.

__Zinc lozenges quicken the immune response__ and aid in reducing an ear infection. __Beta-carotene and vitamin E__ promotes healing of the mucous membranes. Wash your hands. This is the single best way to prevent the spread of illness.

When using eardrops, be sure to treat both ears even if the infection appears only in one ear. Sleep with the head propped up to relieve pressure on the eardrum and promote drainage. Avoid all fast and convenience foods: think of these as empty calories, since they tend to be low in needed nutrients.

Daily eucalyptus inhalation can loosen mucus. To steaming water, add three drops __eucalyptus oil__. Have the child lean over the steam with a towel covering the head, breathing in the inhalation. Put hygroscopic anhydrous glycerin into the ear. Sugar and refined white flour rob the body of potassium and phosphorus, which are critical to preventing and treating ear function.

ECZEMA / DERMATITIS: Eczema or atopic dermatitis is a form of dermatitis, or inflammation of the epidermis (the outer layer of the skin) that is usually chronic. The term eczema is broadly applied to a range of persistent skin conditions (rashes). Eczema and dermatitis are essentially the same. There are many types of dermatitis.

The skin is the largest organ of the body, with a total area of about 20 square feet. The skin protects us from microbes and the elements: it helps regulate body temperature: and permits the sensations of touch, heat, and cold. Skin has three layers: The epidermis, the outermost layer of skin, provides a waterproof barrier and creates our skin tone. The dermis, beneath the epidermis, contains tough connective tissue, hair follicles, and sweat glands. The deeper subcutaneous tissue (hypodermis) is made of fat and connective tissue. The skin's color is created by special cells called melanocytes, which produce the pigment melanin. Melanocytes are located in the epidermis.

Signs and Symptoms: dryness and recurring skin rashes that are characterized by one or more of these symptoms: redness, skin edema (swelling), itching and dryness, crusting, flaking, bumps, blistering, cracking, oozing, or bleeding. Areas of temporary skin discoloration may appear and are sometimes due to healed injuries. Scratching open a healing lesion may result in scarring and may enlarge the rash.

Causes of eczema is unknown, but is presumed to be a combination of genetic and environmental factors. Researchers have compared the prevalence of eczema in people who also suffer from celiac disease to eczema prevalence in control subjects, and they've found that eczema occurs about three times more frequently in celiac disease patients and about two times more frequently in relatives of celiac patients, potentially indicating a genetic link.

Nutritional factors: Recent studies provide hints that food allergy may trigger most forms of dermatitis. For these people, identifying the allergens could lead to an avoidance diet to help minimize symptoms, although this approach is still in an experimental stage.

Dietary triggers include: dairy products, fish, soybean products, eggs, nuts, wheat gluten and maize: however, food allergies may vary from person to person. Studies suggest that use of oral vitamin D3 supplements bolsters production of a protective chemical normally found in the skin, and may help prevent skin irritations that are a common result of atopic dermatitis, the most common form of eczema.

A number of alternative therapies are used for eczema including: Sulfur has been used for many years as a topical treatment in the alleviation of eczema. Probiotics are live microorganisms such as the Lactobacillus bacteria found in yogurt. They are not effective for treating eczema in older populations, but some research points to some strains of beneficial microorganisms having the ability to prevent the following **triad:** allergies, atopic dermatitis and asthma.

Specific nutrients - that aid in prevention and/or recovery of most forms of dermatitis are: chromium, selenium, zinc, Vitamins A and E and foods that contain sulfur i.e., onions, leeks, scallions, and garlic. Zinc plays a vital role in the production and action of many hormones as well as plays a significant role in wound healing, the immune response, and tissue regeneration. Foods rich in zinc are nuts, seeds, whole grains, and legumes. Also, dietary antioxidants high in Vitamin A and E, such as fruits and vegetables.

Behavioral approach. Patients can undergo a six-week monitored program involving scratch habit reversal and self-awareness of scratching levels. For long-term eczema sufferers, scratching can become habitual. Sometimes scratching becomes a reflex, resulting in scratching without conscious awareness, rather than from the feeling of itchiness itself. Complex eczema / dermatitis can be treated with antifungal-and-corticosteroid combination creams.

FIBROCYSTIC BREAST DISEASE: Fibrocystic Breast Disease (Also called fibrocystic condition, fibrocystic change or cystic mastitis). Fibrocystic breast disease is more a characteristic of the breast than a disease. Fibrocystic changes are often more prominent during ovulation and just before menstruation.

Hormone level changes often cause the breast cells to retain fluid and develop into nodules or cysts (fluid filled sacs), which feel like a lump when touched. Fluid filled cysts or lumps is what is known as fibrocyctic breast disease. The nodules or cysts can spread throughout the breast, may be located in one general area or simply appear as one or more large cysts. If the lump is not filled with fluid, it is called a fibroadenoma. A fibroadenoma is a solitary, firm distinct lump, composed of a mass or lump of fibrous tissue.

Signs and Symptoms: Signs and symptoms of fibrocystic breast disease are: tenderness in one or both breasts with pressure or touch, breast pain, an intermittent or persistent sense of breast engorgement, associated with dull, heavy pain and tenderness, intermittent appearance of cysts or lumps that form and then resolve within a few weeks, a dense, pebbly consistency to breast tissue, formation of persistent cysts or lumps, nipple discharge or inflammation. These symptoms can range from mild to severe. Many women notice monthly cyclic patterns, with symptoms most severe just before each menstrual period. *Having fibrocystic breasts does not place women at a higher or lower risk of developing breast cancer.*

Causes: of fibrocystic breast condition is not actually known for sure, however the symptoms and signs are linked to a woman's hormone patterns and diet. Each month, the breasts respond to the cyclic peaks and troughs of estrogen and progesterone. As hormone levels rise just before and during menstruation, mammary blood vessels swell, ducts and alveoli expand, and cell growth proliferates and breast tissue retains fluid and grows larger. After menstruation, these processes reverse. Years of such fluctuations eventually produce areas of dense or fibrotic tissue.

Multiple small cysts and an increasing level of breast pain commonly develop when a woman hits her 30s. Larger cysts usually do not occur until after the age of 35. Fibrocystic breast disease is usually diagnosed when a patient goes to her doctor for a checkup or seeks help for pain, tenderness or a lump that was probably discovered during breast self-examination.

The doctor will examine the breasts and sometimes recommend a mammogram, an ultrasound exam and (rarely) a needle aspiration. Most of the time the diagnosis of fibrocystic breast characteristics does not require extensive testing. Needle aspiration involves inserting a needle into the middle of the lump to see whether it's a mass of tissue or a fluid-filled cyst. If the lump does not yield fluid when aspirated, it may still be a cyst or other benign growth, such as intraductal papilloma (warty growth), fat necrosis (a fatty lump), duct ectasia (a clogged mammary duct) or sclerosing adenosis (a calcium deposit). Ultrasound will determine if it is a simple cyst.

If the cyst is not normal in appearance, does not disappear with aspiration or recurs after repeated aspiration, the doctor may do a biopsy to check for possible cancer. A biopsy involves removing all or part of the lump and examining it for cancer. There are needle biopsies (removing cells), incisional biopsies (surgical removal of only part of the lump) and excisional biopsies (removing all of the lump).

During the examination of the lump sample, the pathologist might see excessive fibrous growth between the breast glands or cyst formation within the glands. This condition is called atypical hyperplasia. Atypical hyperplasia is associated with a fivefold increase in breast cancer risk and is found in an estimated 4 to 10 percent of women with lumpy breasts. There are no specific treatments for fibrocystic breast disease, other than those to minimize discomfort. Doctors may recommend the following: wear a firm bra that gives very good support for severe breast pain.

Nutritional factors: avoid caffeine and chocolate: and eliminate excessive dietary fat, especially trans-fats , i.e., hydrogenated oils, and limit salt and sugar intake. Take **fish oil** capsules 1,000 mg two to three times a day along with pain relievers for combating pain and inflammation and increase doses of **vitamin E**. Ingesting **more natural foods with anti-oxidants and anti-inflammatory nutrients** (raw fruit and vegetables, pg 183) as well as reducing or eliminating those food products containing bad fats, (hydrogenated oils), sugars and artificial nonnutritive sweeteners will help prevent as well as treat this disease.

FIBROMYALGIA: **(SEE CHRONIC FATIGUE SYNDROME/POLYMYALGIA RHEUMATICA)**

FOOD ALLERGIES: **(SEE ALLERGIES)**

GALLSTONES: The gallbladder is a small sac located in the abdomen below the liver. Gallstones are formed when liquid (bile) that is stored in the gallbladder hardens into small pebble-like pieces. There are two types of gallstones--those made of cholesterol and those composed of bilirubin. Cholesterol stones are the most common type of gallstones. Gallstones can block the normal flow of bile, causing severe pain and even death if untreated.

Signs and Symptoms: Pain is the upper right corner of the abdomen radiating to the back beneath the shoulder bone (scapula) and sometimes associated with nausea.

Causes of Gallstones: gallstones made of cholesterol are thought to be caused by: too much cholesterol and the combination of too much bilirubin and not enough bile salts. The rate and degree at which the gallbladder empties is also a contributing factor. The causes of pigment stones are not fully understood.

Nutritional factors: Diets high in fat and cholesterol and low in fiber is the major cause the formation of gallstones. Eggs, dairy products and fatty meats should be eaten in moderation. Individuals should opt for lean meats such as turkey, chicken or seafood. Frying and sautéing are methods that result in higher levels of fat. Boiling, steaming and baking are options for cooking that can reduce fat and cholesterol without sacrificing flavor.

Diets low in fiber can also contribute to the development of gallstones. **Fiber** helps regulate the digestive system and allows bile to move through the system quicker. Fiber is found in a large variety of food sources.

Raw fruits and vegetables are excellent sources of dietary fiber. Brown rice and whole-grain options will also increase fiber. Beans are a great source of fiber that can be included in a wide variety of dishes. The gallbladder plays an important role in the digestion of foods. Being overweight can increase the likelihood of gallstones: although adopting a low-fat diet may lead to weight loss. Clear liquids provide the digestive system much needed rest and can often allow the gallstones to pass if small enough.

GASTROESOPHAGEAL REFLUX DISEASE: (GERD), (aka, Non-ulcer Dyspepsia, Gastric Reflux Disease, or Acid Reflux Disease or Heartburn) Gastroesophageal reflux disease is a chronic symptom of mucosal damage caused by stomach acid coming up from the stomach into the esophagus. GERD is usually caused by changes in the barrier between the stomach and the esophagus, including abnormal relaxation of the lower esophageal sphincter, which normally holds the top of the stomach closed: impaired expulsion of gastric reflux from the esophagus: or a hiatyl hernia. These changes may be permanent or temporary ("transient").

Another kind of acid reflux, which causes respiratory and laryngeal signs and symptoms, is called laryngpharyngeal reflux (LPR) or "extra-esophageal reflux disease" (EERD). Unlike GERD, LPR rarely produces heartburn, and is sometimes called silent reflux. However, it can cause hoarseness.

The function of the stomach is to generate strong acids (HCl) and enzymes (such as pepsin) to aid in food digestion. This digestive mixture is called gastric juice. The inner lining of the stomach has several mechanisms to resist the effect of gastric juice on itself, but the mucosa of the esophagus does not.

The esophagus is normally protected from these acids by a one-way valve mechanism at its junction with the stomach. This one-way valve is called the esophageal sphincter (ES), and this sphincter prevents gastric juice from flowing back into the esophagus. During peristalsis, the ES allows the food bolus to pass into the stomach. It prevents chyme, a mixture of bolus, stomach acid, and digestive enzymes, from returning up the esophagus.

The ES is aided in the task of keeping the flow of materials in one direction. The ES is a functional sphincter but not an anatomical sphincter: that is to say, though there is no thickening of the smooth muscle, as in the pyloric sphincter. Chyme is (usually) prevented from travelling back from the stomach up the esophagus by this sphincter. The lower muscles in the esophagus help this sphincteric action.

Treating Acid Reflux (GERD) Naturally: There are many ways to treat acid reflux which include making some lifestyle changes, avoiding certain foods and even utilizing some natural options for healing and suppression of symptoms. One of the most important things you can do in the natural treatment of acid reflux is to make some dietary adjustments. You can and need to learn which foods to avoid and which ones will actually reduce acid build up and aid your digestive system.

Foods to Avoid with Acid Reflux are: *Avoid tomatoes, oranges, grapefruits and lemons along with the juices of these fruits, including lemonade and cranberry juice. You should also stay away from tomato products like tomato sauce, red spaghetti sauce, catsup, etc.

*There are many vegetables which can exacerbate acid reflux. These include mashed potatoes, and especially French fries. You should also avoid garlic, chilies and hot peppers. *Meat Products to avoid include: hamburger that is not designated as lean or extra-lean, chicken products like nuggets, fried chicken and any prepared meats with fat and spice like Buffalo wings. Fish with a high fat content like salmon and marbled meats like sirloin should also be avoided.

*Dairy products like regular sour cream, cottage cheese, milk shakes or ice cream can exacerbate acid reflux. *Avoid spaghetti with red sauce and macaroni and cheese. *There are many beverages to avoid. *Wine can really cause acid reflux as can other liquors. So can decaffeinated or regular coffee or tea. *Peppermint tea can cause the valve between the esophagus and the stomach to relax, which allows the reflux of stomach contents into the throat. *Chocolate will also cause this valve to relax and should be avoided. *Cookies, doughnuts, corn chips and brownies, etc., can also cause acid reflux.

Foods to Combat Acid Reflux are: Many foods are considered neutral, meaning they won't trigger acid reflux and some will actually prevent the build-up of acid. These neutral foods include: apples and bananas which are both great options fresh, dried or as juices.

Mineral water can actually help neutralize acid so it is a great choice of beverage. Vegetables include broccoli and baked potatoes, carrots, green beans and peas. Lean meats won't exacerbate symptoms. Choose lean hamburger, chicken breast without the skin, egg whites, lean varieties of fish and broiled steak.

Fat-free versions of cream cheese, sour cream, yogurt and goat or soy cheese are good choices. Oatmeal, bran and other cereal grains, brown and white rice, white or multi-grain bread, rice cakes, any graham cookies and also corn bread or pretzels. Other items like low-fat salad dressing, fat-free cookies, baked varieties of crackers or potato chips and sweets like licorice or jelly beans, won't aggravate acid reflux.

Lifestyle Do's and Don'ts for Acid Reflux. *Don't drink wine or beer several hours before going to bed. You may have to cut it out all together because - wine can cause acid reflux and beer can increase the amount of acid in your stomach to two times the normal amount within an hour.

*If you need to drink something before bed, your best choice is water or apple juice. If you already have heartburn before you go to bed, drinking apple juice or eating an apple will really help reduce the amount of acid you have in your stomach. *Do drink water throughout the day. It will help dilute stomach acid and help minimize heartburn. You should also drink one or two glasses after every meal and a small glass of water before you go to bed.

*Don't eat for three or four hours before you go to bed. *Eat four to six small meals throughout the day instead of three larger ones. Take time with each meal, chew your food and relax. *Being overweight can exacerbate and even cause acid reflux. Losing even a few pounds can make a big impact on reducing symptoms. *Don't drink peppermint tea or eat peppermint or chocolate candy as it relaxes the sphincter (ES).

Nutritional info. There are some great natural treatments for acid reflux, including: Ginger in any form can reduce acid reflux. Candied ginger, ginger tea, ginger supplements, <u>real ginger ale</u> and any other type are great ways to combat heartburn and acid reflux. Chewing an apple or a couple of <u>almonds</u> before and/or after each meal can help eliminate acid reflux if you chew them thoroughly.

Chamomile tea can soothe the digestive system, including the stomach. One of the best natural treatments for acid reflux is to mix a half a cup of organic apple cider vinegar with a half a cup of water, drinking it right before or right after a meal. <u>This remedy also helps in weight loss diets.</u>

GINGIVITIS : **(SEE ALSO PERIODONTAL DISEASE)** Gingivitis is "inflammation of the gum tissue". The most common form of gingivitis, and the most common form of periodontal disease overall is in response to bacterial biofilms (also called plaque) which adherent to tooth surfaces, termed <u>plaque-induced gingivitis</u>. In the absence of treatment, gingivitis may progress to <u>periodontitis,</u> which is a destructive form of periodontal disease. While in some sites or individuals, gingivitis never progresses to periodontitis. Data indicates that periodontitis is always preceded by gingivitis.

Signs and Symptoms: The symptoms of gingivitis are somewhat non-specific and manifest in the gum tissue as the classic signs of inflammation: Swollen gums: Bright red or purple gum: Gums that are tender or painful to the touch: Bleeding gums or bleeding after brushing. Additionally, the stippling that normally exists on the gum tissue will often disappear and the gums may appear shiny when the gum tissue becomes swollen and stretched over the inflamed underlying connective tissue. The accumulation may also emit an unpleasant odor. When the gingiva are swollen, the epithelial lining of the gingival crevice becomes ulcerated and the gums will bleed more easily with even gentle brushing, and especially when flossing.

Cause: <u>plaque-induced gingivitis</u> is by far the most common form of gingival diseases. The etiology, or cause, of plaque-induced gingivitis is bacterial plaque, which acts to initiate the body's host response. This, in turn, can lead to destruction of the gingival tissues, which may progress to destruction of the periodontal attachment apparatus. The plaque accumulates in the small gaps between teeth, in the gingival grooves and in areas known as plaque traps (locations that serve to accumulate and maintain plaque). Examples of plaque traps include bulky and overhanging restorative margins, claps of removable partial dentures and calculus (tartar) that forms on teeth. Although these accumulations may be tiny, the bacteria in them produce chemicals, such as degradative enzymes and toxins that promote an inflammatory response in the gum tissue. This inflammation can cause inflammation and plaque.

Nutritional Factors: You can help prevent and combat gingivitis with food. There are certain foods that combat gingivitis by minimizing the build-up of bacteria. Eat firm crunchy natural foods. Crunchy foods such as celery and apples help to remove food particles that may stick to the teeth. Soft foods, such as chocolate and peanut butter, for example, tent to get stuck in the crevices between the teeth. Food that gets stuck helps to promote bacterial growth and increase the chances of developing gingivitis.

Get ample amounts of fiber. While the fiber doesn't directly take the bacteria away from your teeth to reduce the chances of getting gingivitis, what fiber does is it helps to improve your body's immune system. Fiber rich foods such as whole grains, fruits, beans and vegetables provide the necessary building blocks for a healthy immune system which places your body in a better position to fight bacteria that causes gingivitis.

Stay away from sugars. Sugar on the teeth is like a Thanksgiving meal for bacteria. Bacteria thrive on sugar left on and in between the teeth. If you feel that you cannot give up sugar entirely, make sure to brush your teeth afterward.

Treatment. Therapy is aimed at the reduction of oral bacteria, and may take the form of regular periodic visits to a dental professional together with adequate oral hygiene home care. Thus, several of the methods used in the prevention of gingivitis can also be used for the treatment of manifest gingivitis, such as scaling, root planning, curettage, mouth washes containing chlorhexidine or hydrogen peroxide, and flossing. Inter-dental brushes also help remove any causative agents. Recent scientific studies have also shown the beneficial effects of mouthwashes with essential oils.

GLAUCOMA: Glaucoma is a <u>disease of the optic nerve</u>, the major nerve of vision. The optic nerve receives light-generated nerve impulses from the retina and transmits these to the brain, where we recognize those electrical signals as vision. Glaucoma is characterized by a particular pattern of progressive damage to the optic nerve that generally <u>begins with a subtle loss of side vision (peripheral vision)</u>.

If glaucoma is not diagnosed and treated, it can progress to loss of central vision and blindness. Glaucoma is usually, but not always, associated with elevated pressure in the eye (intraocular pressure). Generally, it is this elevated eye pressure that leads to damage of the eye (optic) nerve. In some cases, glaucoma may occur in the presence of normal eye pressure. This form of glaucoma is believed to be caused by poor regulation of blood flow to the optic nerve. Glaucoma is the leading cause of irreversible blindness.

Signs and Symptoms: Glaucoma <u>initially causes no symptoms</u>, and the subsequent loss of side vision (peripheral vision) is usually not recognized until too late.

Causes: Elevated pressure in the eye is the main factor leading to glaucomatous damage to the eye (optic) nerve. This nerve transmits the images we see back to the brain for interpretation. The eye is firm and round, like a basketball. Its tone and shape are maintained by a pressure within the eye (the intraocular pressure), which normally ranges between 8 mm and 22 mm (millimeters) of mercury. When the pressure is too low, the eye becomes softer, while an elevated pressure causes the eye to become harder.

The optic nerve is the most susceptible part of the eye to high pressure because the delicate fibers in this nerve are easily damaged. The cornea covers the iris and the pupil, which are in front of the lens. The pupil is the small, round, black-appearing opening in the center of the iris. Light passes through the pupil, on through the lens, and to the retina at the back of the eye.

The front of the eye is filled with a clear fluid called the aqueous humor, which provides nourishment to the structures in the front of the eye. This fluid is produced constantly by the ciliary body, which surrounds the lens of the eye. The aqueous humor then flows through the pupil and leaves the eye through tiny channels called the trabecular meshwork. These channels are located at what is called the drainage angle of the eye. This angle is where the clear cornea, which covers the front of the eye, attaches to the base of the iris, which is the colored part of the eye. In most people, the drainage angles are wide open, although in some individuals, they can be narrow. For example, the usual angle is about 45 degrees, whereas a narrow angle is about 25 degrees or less.

After exiting through the trabecular meshwork in the drainage angle, the aqueous fluid then drains into tiny blood vessels (capillaries) into the main bloodstream. The aqueous humor should not be confused with tears, which are produced by a gland outside of the eyeball itself. If too much fluid is being produced within the eye, the intraocular pressure may become too high. In either event, since the eye is a closed system, if it cannot remove the increased fluid, the pressure builds up and optic-nerve damage may result causing glaucoma.

Nutritional factors: Spinach contains high amounts of the antioxidants lutein and zeaxanthin which are nutrients that are found in high amounts in your eyes. It is believed that these two nutrients may be important for protecting your eyes against some of the bad effects that can be caused by oxidation. That's why they are called antioxidants. Eating more spinach and other green leafy vegetables and/or taking supplements rich in antioxidants will help with all kinds of problems, including cataracts and glaucoma. Carrots are high in beta-carotene, also an antioxidant found in the eye. There are also other nutrients thought to be good for protecting vision because of their antioxidant abilities, including **vitamins A, C, E** and the mineral **zinc**.

List of Foods High In Antioxidants (Also see Appendix for complete list)

Vitamin A: Liver, Egg yolks, Whole milk, Cheese, Carrots, Sweet potato, Kale, Broccoli, Turnip greens, Mustard greens, Beet greens, Collard greens, Red peppers, Pink Grapefruit, Cantaloupe, Apricots, Papaya.
Vitamin C: Citrus fruits (oranges grapefruit, lemons), Berries, Tomatoes, Peppers, Cabbage, Broccoli, Brussels Sprouts, Cauliflower, Cantaloupe
Vitamin E: Vegetable oils (wheat germ oil is especially rich in vitamin E), Wheat-germ and other Whole grains, Green leafy vegetables, Egg yolk, Milk fat, Butter, Unprocessed Meat, Nuts, Organ Meats (liver), Seafood, Avocados.
Zinc: Lean meat, Seafood, (especially oysters and shrimp), Eggs, Green leafy vegetables, Soybeans, Peanuts and Peanut butter, Whole Bran, Whole grain cereals (especially oatmeal), Cheese.
Lutein and Zeaxanthin: Kale, Collard greens, Spinach, Parsley (not dried), Celery, Broccoli, Lettuce, Green peas, Pumpkin, Brussels sprouts, Summer squash, Corn, Green beans, Green peppers, Cucumbers, Green olives.

GOUT: Gout (also known as podagra when it involves the big toe) is a medical condition usually characterized by recurrent attacks of acute inflammatory arthritis, i.e., <u>a red, tender, hot, swollen joint</u>. The metatarsal-phalangeal joint at the base of the big toe is the most commonly affected (approximately 50% of cases). However, it may also present as tophi, kidney stones, or urate nephropathy. It is caused by elevated levels of uric acid in the blood which crystallize, and the crystals are deposited in joints, tendons, and surrounding tissues. A clinical diagnosis is confirmed by the visualization of the characteristic crystals in joint fluid. <u>Gout is often acquired through the foods and beverages a person consumes</u>. These foods are the reason why the uric acid level of the body increases. Uric acid normally dissolves in the blood but trouble comes in when the amount exceeds its normal production. They can't be suspended, thus they form needle-like crystals in the joints. This formation of crystals is termed "gout". Gout attacks can give excruciating pain that may prevent victims to do any work or even move. Gout has increased in frequency in recent decades, affecting about 1-2% of the Western population at some point in their lives. The increase is believed to be due to increasing risk factors in the population, such as metabolic syndrome, longer life expectancy and changes in diet. Historically, gout was known as "the disease of kings" or "rich man's disease".

Signs and Symptoms: Gout can present in a number of ways, although the most usual is a recurrent attack of acute <u>inflammatory arthritis</u> (a red, tender, hot, swollen joint). The metatarsal-phalangeal joint at the base of the <u>big toe</u> is affected most often, accounting for half of cases. Other joints, such as the heels, knees, wrists and fingers, may also be affected. Joint pain usually begins over 2–4 hours and during the night. The reason for onset at night is due to the lower body temperature. Other symptoms may occur along with the joint pain, including <u>fatigue</u> and a high <u>fever</u>. Long-

125

standing elevated <u>uric acid</u> levels may result (hyperuricemia) in other symptomatology, including hard, painless deposits of uric acid crystals known as <u>tophi</u>. Extensive tophi may lead to chronic <u>arthritis</u> due to bone erosion. Elevated levels of uric acid may also lead to crystals precipitating in the <u>kidneys</u>, resulting in <u>stone</u> formation and subsequent <u>urate nephropathy</u>.

Cause: <u>Hyperuricemia</u> is the underlying cause of gout. This can occur for a number of reasons, including diet, genetic predisposition, or underexcretion of <u>urate</u>, the salts of uric acid. Renal under-excretion of uric acid is the primary cause of hyperuricemia in about 90% of cases, while overproduction is the cause in less than 10%. About 10% of people with hyperuricemia develop gout at some point in their lifetimes. The risk, however, varies depending on the degree of hyperuricemia.

<u>Dietary</u>: causes account for about 12% of gout, and include a strong association with the consumption of alcohol, <u>fructose</u>-sweetened soda and juice drinks, processed meats, and seafood. Other triggers include <u>physical trauma</u> and surgery.

<u>Genetics</u>: The occurrence of gout is partly genetic, contributing to about 60% of <u>variability</u> in uric acid level. Two <u>genes</u> called <u>SLC2A9</u> and <u>ABCG2</u> have been found to commonly be associated with gout, and variations in them can approximately double the risk. A few rare genetic disorders, including familial juvenile hyperuricemic nephropathy, phosphoribosylpyrophosphate synthetase superactivity, medullary cystic kidney disease, and hypoxanthine-guanine phosphoribosyltransferase deficiency as seen in Lesch-Nyhan syndrome, are complicated by gout.

<u>Medical conditions</u>: Gout frequently occurs in combination with other medical problems. For example, <u>the Metabolic syndrome</u>, which is a combination of abdominal obesity, hypertension, insulin resistance and abnormal lipid levels, occurs in nearly 75% of cases.

Other conditions commonly complicated by gout include: polycythemia, lead poisoning, renal failure, hemolytic anemia, psoriasis, and solid organ transplants. A body mass index greater than or equal to 35 increases a male's risk of gout threefold. Chronic lead exposure and lead-contaminated alcohol are risk factors for gout due to the harmful effect of lead on kidney function. Lesch-Nyhan syndrome is often associated with gouty arthritis. Medication: Diuretics have been associated with attacks of gout. However, a low dose of hydrochlorothiazide does not seem to increase the risk. Other medicines that have been associated include niacin, and acetylsalicylic acid (aspirin) . The immunosuppressive drugs ciclosporin is also associated with gout, when used in combination with hydrochlorothiazide, a fluid pill.

Nutritional factors: Since food is one of the factors that brings on this condition, it is only appropriate to provide the best diet for gout sufferers that can help them prevent having any attacks. Foods that are high in purine are not considered best diet for gout sufferers. In fact, they should be abandoned completely. Purine is broken down by the body into uric acid, which is the reason why the uric acid level rises so fast if a person takes in purine-rich food. Examples of these are sardines, organ meat, processed meats, like bologna, anchovies, scallops, meat extracts, and mackerel.

On the other hand, **eating 10-15 cherries- daily is one of the best diets** for gout sufferers as it contains enzymes and anti-inflammatory compounds that can help balance uric acid level. This will lessen the occurrence of gout attacks besides its delicious taste. Not only that, it also encourages excretion of uric acid through urination. Cherries work in the same way with vitamin C. It is loaded with natural fibers but low in calorie content. Cherries are anti-inflammatory and can also lessen the amount of CRP (C-Reactive Protein) which is an inflammatory chemical found in the blood of individuals with heart disease, gout, and diabetes.

Both **sweet** and **sour cherries** are full of <u>vitamin A and antioxidants</u>, which decongests arteries and tissue blocked by uric acid crystals. **Garlic and ginger** are spices that <u>should be included</u> in the foods of gout victims for they are known to be good in decreasing uric acid level of the body, which prevents frequent gout attacks. <u>Lack of potassium </u>can lead to increase in the amount of uric acid. Eating **banana** and other foods rich in potassium <u>ease inflammation</u> and gout attacks. Having bananas daily is good for gout patients.

Other foods that can be source of potassium are <u>potatoes, beans, vegetables and other fruits</u>. Low fat dairy products, complex carbohydrates, green leafy vegetables, and fresh fruits are also considered best diet for gout sufferers. These foods can prevent gout attacks, making them ideal for the victims. The consumption of beans, peas, lentils, and spinach, lean protein, coffee, vitamin C and dairy products, as well as physical fitness, appear to decrease the risk. This is believed to be partly due to their effect in reducing insulin resistance. Above all, drinking a lot of pure water regularly will help neutralize the body's uric acid level. So, it is always recommended to have at least 8-10 glasses of natural non-flavored water daily.

Treatment: Pharmacologically nonsteroidal anti-inflammatory drugs (NSAIDs), steroids, especially indomethacin (Indocin) and/or colchicine is the main stay. These drugs improve symptoms. Once the acute attack has subsided, levels of uric acid are usually lowered via lifestyle changes, and in those with frequent attacks, allopurinol or probenecid provide long-term prevention.

HAY FEVER: **SEE ALLERGIC RHINITIS**

HEADACHE: **(MIGRAINE AND NONMIGRAINE OR TENSION)** A headache or cephalalgia is pain anywhere in the region of the head or neck. It can be a symptom of a number of different conditions of the head and neck. <u>However, the brain tissue itself is not sensitive</u>

to pain because it lacks pain receptors. Rather, the pain is caused by disturbance of the pain-sensitive structures around the brain. Nine areas of the head and neck have these pain-sensitive structures. They are the cranium (the periosteum of the skull), muscles, nerves, arteries and veins, subcutaneous tissues, sinuses, eyes, ears, and mucous membranes. Headache is a response of nociceptive areas of scalp and brain to any external or internal stimulus that causes pain.

Signs, Symptoms and Causes: There are thousands of causes of headache. Each and every cause can produce headache in different magnitudes. Headache can be transient or it may be persistent. It may be trivial in case of external injury or may be severe in case of a migraine attack. Pain killers are good to treat any episode of headache, but many produce severe or bad side effects, i.e., gastritis, kidney and liver disease.

Since there are over 200 types of headache, and the causes range from harmless to life-threatening it is important to determine the cause or precipitating factor(s). And the description of the headache, together with findings on neurological examination, will determine the need for any further investigations and the most appropriate treatment. Basically there are two main categories of headaches: primary headaches and secondary headaches.

Primary headaches. The most common types of headache are the "primary headache disorders", such as tension-type headache and migraine. They have typical features: migraine, for example, tends to be pulsating in character, affecting one side of the head, associated with nausea, disabling in severity, and usually lasts between 3 hours and 3 days. Rarer primary headache disorders are trigeminal neuralgia (a shooting face pain), cluster headache (severe pains that occur together in bouts), and hemi-cranial continua (a continuous headache on one side of the head).

Secondary headaches. Headaches may be caused by problems elsewhere in the head or neck. Some of these are not harmful, such as cervicogenic headache (pain arising from the neck muscles). A number of characteristics make it more likely that the headache is due to potentially dangerous secondary causes: some of these may be life-threatening or cause long-term damage.

A number of "red flag" symptoms therefore means that a headache warrants further investigations, usually by a specialist. The red flag symptoms are a new or different headache in someone over 50 years old, headache that develops within minutes (thunderclap headache), inability to move a limb or abnormalities on neurological examination, mental confusion, being woken by headache, headache that worsens with changing posture, headache worsened by exertion or Valsalva maneuver (coughing, straining), visual loss or visual abnormalities, jaw claudication (jaw pain on chewing that resolves afterwards), neck stiffness, fever, and headaches in people with HIV, cancer or risk factors for thrombosis.

A "thunderclap headache" may be the only symptom of subarachnoid hemorrhage, a form of stroke in which blood accumulates around the brain, often from a ruptured brain aneurysm. Headache with fever may be caused by meningitis, particularly if there is meningism (inability to flex the neck forward due to stiffness), and confusion may be indicative of encephalitis (inflammation of the brain, usually due to particular viruses).

Headache that is worsened by straining or a change in position may be caused by increased pressure in the skull: this is often worse in the morning and associated with vomiting. Raised intracranial pressure may be due to brain tumors, and idiopathic intracranial hypertension, more common in overweight women, and occasionally cerebral venous sinus thrombosis. Headache together with weakness in part of the body may indicate a stroke (particularly intracranial hemorrhage or subdural hematoma) or brain tumor.

Headache in older people, particularly when associated with visual symptoms or jaw claudication, may indicate giant cell arteritis (GCA), in which the blood vessel wall is inflamed and obstructs blood flow. Carbon monoxide poisoning may lead to headaches as well as nausea, vomiting, dizziness, muscle weakness and blurred vision. Angle closure glaucoma (acute raised pressure in the eyeball) may lead to headache, particularly around the eye, as well as visual abnormalities, nausea, vomiting and a red eye with a dilated pupil.

Nutritional cures: can be ideal if any person suffers from recurrent bouts of headache. The 10 best foods known to cure headaches.

Water: this is the cheapest and may be most reliable food to cure headache. If your body is properly hydrated, most of the toxins will be flushed out through urine, stool or sweat. Water also helps regulate the temperature of our body through a complex mechanism in the brain stem.

Coffee: a strong cup of coffee, can help you if you are suffering from severe headache. Coffee contains caffeine and it contracts the small blood vessels in the cranium. Thus the nerve endings which initiate the sense of pain also get hypo-stimulated.

Tea: contains tannin. For the same reason, a strong cup of tea will also cure headache.

Ginkgo biloba: is a medicinal plant. The leaves and the seeds contain some flavonoid glycosides. Clinical trials have strongly recommended use of ginkgo biloba in those patients suffering from dementia and chronic headache.

Banana: if you suffer from constant headache, you should include a banana in your breakfast every day. High magnesium concentration in bananas will help in the successful cure of headache. Lemonade: a glass of lemonade or fresh lime juice with high concentration of salt can cure severe headache almost instantly. Intake of salt is not generally prescribed, but in case of headache, it acts like magic.

Apple: denuded and seed free pieces of apples, each morning in your breakfast will definitely cure stress related headache. Apples contain bioflavonoids which help in reduction of blood pressure and thus reducing the incidence of headache.

Black pepper: either in powdered form or mixed with vegetables, it can cure headache. Black pepper contains capsaicin and it can increase the threshold level for headache.

Herbal infusion drink containing lots of antioxidants: Mix some basil leaves and ginger pieces in boiling water. Let it boil for 5-7 minutes. Sift the water into a cup. Add 1 tsp of honey. Drink it warm. You will feel better. Selenium, magnesium and vitamins will help your body to rejuvenate instantly. Milk: warm milk has a soothing effect over our nervous system. For a nagging headache, you can take a glassful of milk with added real sugar. Along with these 10 foods, adequate rest and proper nutrition, you can actually reduce markedly the incidence of one of the most irritating diseases of our body.

Summary: One thing for certain that will trigger a headache quicker than anything is "not eating". **Food "triggers"** may include these: Alcohol, specifically red wine, but also other beverages, even herbal teas, Aspartame sweetener, Beans and other tyramine-containing foods, Cheeses and yogurt, Chinese food or other soups and foods containing MSG, Chocolate, Processed meats (containing sulfites-egg, bacon, sausages, salami, ham).

There are many foods that are considered **"safe" foods** which shouldn't "trigger" pain. These include: <u>Rice</u>, especially brown rice, <u>Cooked green vegetables</u>, such as broccoli, kale, spinach, Swiss chard, or collards, <u>Cooked orange vegetables</u>, such as carrots or sweet potatoes, <u>Cooked yellow vegetables</u>, such as summer squash, <u>Cooked or dried non-citrus fruits</u>: cherries, pears, prunes (but not bananas, peaches, tomatoes). <u>Water</u>: Plain water or carbonated forms, such as Perrier, are fine. Condiments: Modest amounts of salt, maple syrup, and vanilla extract are usually well-tolerated.

Summary of foods that can prevent or treat most headaches are: bananas, apples, pears, warm milk, unsalted nuts, coffee and tea without sugar (you may use honey to sweeten - a little), lemon or lime juice, ginger capsules, ginger tea, red or black pepper. Also any natural unprocessed food that contains noteworthy amounts of selenium, magnesium, vitamins A, B, C, and even D can prevent or treat most headaches.

HEARTBURN: **(SEE GASTROESOPHAGEAL REFLUX DISEASE)**

HEART DISEASE: **(SEE ATHEROSCLEROSIS OR CHOLESTEROL DISORDER)**

HEMORRHOIDS: Hemorrhoids are vascular structures in the anal canal which help with stool control. They become pathological or "piles" when swollen or inflamed. In their physiological state, they act as a cushion composed of arterio-venous channels and connective tissue that aid the passage of stool. There are two types of hemorrhoids, <u>external</u> and <u>internal</u>, which are differentiated via their position with respect to the dentate line. External hemorrhoids are those that occur below the dentate or pectinate line. Specifically, they are varicosities of the veins draining the territory of the inferior rectal arteries, which are branches of the internal pudendal artery.

Signs and Symptoms: Hemorrhoids are sometimes painful, and are often accompanied by swelling, irritation and/or itching. Itching, although often thought to be a symptom of external hemorrhoids, is more commonly due to skin irritation. The skin irritation may be brought about by the inflammation of the external hemorrhoid which in turn leads to a barely noticeable watery discharge and skin irritation.

External hemorrhoids are prone to thrombosis: if the vein ruptures and/or a blood clot develops, the hemorrhoid becomes a thrombosed hemorrhoid. Internal hemorrhoids are those that occur above the dentate line. Specifically, they are varicosities of veins draining the territory of branches of the superior rectal arteries. As this area lacks pain receptors, internal hemorrhoids are usually not painful and most people are not aware that they have them. Internal hemorrhoids, however, may bleed when irritated.

Untreated internal hemorrhoids can lead to two severe forms of hemorrhoids: prolapsed and strangulated hemorrhoids. Prolapsed hemorrhoids are internal hemorrhoids that are so distended that they are pushed outside the anus. If the anal sphincter muscle goes into spasm and traps a prolapsed hemorrhoid outside the anal opening, the supply of blood is cut off, and the hemorrhoid becomes a strangulated hemorrhoid.

The symptoms of pathological hemorrhoids depend on the type present. Internal hemorrhoids usually present with painless rectal bleeding while external hemorrhoids present more with pain in the area of the anus. External Hemorrhoids usually present with itching, rectal pain, and rectal bleeding. Other symptoms include mucous discharge and fecal incontinence. In most cases, symptoms will resolve within a few days.

External hemorrhoids are painful, while internal hemorrhoids usually are not unless they become thrombosed or necrotic. The most common symptom of internal hemorrhoids is bright red blood covering the stool, a condition known as hematochezia, on toilet paper, or in the toilet bowl. They may protrude through the anus. Symptoms of external hemorrhoids include painful swelling and a lump around the anus.

Causes: A number of factors may lead to the formations of hemorrhoids including irregular bowel habits (constipation or diarrhea), certain exercise, heavy lifting, nutrition (low-fiber diet), genetics, pregnancy, increased intra-abdominal pressure (prolonged straining), absence of valves within the hemorrhoidal veins, obesity, sitting for long periods of time and aging. During pregnancy, pressure from the fetus on the abdomen and hormonal changes cause the hemorrhoidal vessels to enlarge. Delivery also leads to increased intra-abdominal pressures. Surgical treatment is rarely needed, as symptoms usually resolve post delivery.

Nutritional factors: A high fiber diet obtained from raw fruits and vegetables is what you need to follow for eliminating and for preventing constipation and a high fiber diet is what you need to prevent and cure hemorrhoids. If you have not been eating a lot of fiber, you need to add fiber slowly to your diet especially if you add it by using bran. If you add fiber to your diet with fruits and vegetables, you can add them freely without much problem.

However, since your stomach will not be used to it, you may experience more gas for a week or two. Juices are good for hemorrhoids but especially dark berry juice mixed with equal parts of apple juice. The berry juices to use are: cherries, blackberries, blueberries. These berries contain "anthocyanins" and "proanthocyanidins" which reduce hemorrhoidal pain and swelling by toning and strengthening the hemorrhoidal veins. Drink at least one glass of this juice mixture each day.

Also, <u>Red and Black Currant Berries</u>: are high in <u>Vitamin C</u>, <u>rutin</u>, and <u>minerals</u>. This makes their juice valuable in clearing hemorrhoids. They also have a small amount of the gamma linoleic fatty acid (GLA), which produce prostaglandins that control body pain. Drink 1 -2 glasses a day of red or black currant berries. <u>Iron foods</u>: help you build up your blood or to keep iron in reserve, if you ever need it.

The best iron foods are: Liver, Kelp, Prunes, Dried apricots, Sunflower seeds, Pistachios, Cashews, Almonds, Sesame seeds, Potatoes (baked), Swiss chard, Raisins, Cooked Broccoli, and Tuna. Also, <u>cantaloupe is one of the best foods</u> you can eat because it has a good source of phytonutrients, vitamins and minerals. It has a high beta-carotene level and has anti-clogging properties. Ginger, Garlic, and Onion, (herbs), should be added to your diet as they break down fibrin that may accumulate in traumatized veins.

<u>Oils:</u> At every meal, use olive oil, flax seed oil, with apple cider vinegar in your salad: Or at the end of each meal take your capsule of fish oil. <u>Fish oil is one of the most important oils to use daily</u>. Use the following foods to help reduce hemorrhoidal bleeding: Dark green leafy vegetables: Blackstrap molasses: and/or Flax seeds which are high in omega-3 oils.

They are also high in fiber. Lima and butter beans are high in iron, which help to build more blood. If you have bleeding hemorrhoids, adding lima beans to your diet would be a good choice. The above info is a good source of home remedies that can give you temporary relief, reduce bleeding, reduce swelling, eliminate itching, and cure or prevent your hemorrhoids.

Other Recommendations: treatment consists of increasing fiber intake, oral fluids to maintain hydration, NSAID analgesics, sitz baths, hemorrhoidal creams and rest. Surgery is reserved for those who fail to improve following these measures.

HERPES SIMPLEX: Herpes simplex (Ancient Greek: herpes, "creeping" or "latent") is a viral disease from the herpes viridae family caused by both Herpes simplex virus type 1 (HSV-1) and type 2 (HSV-2). Infection with the herpes virus is categorized into one of several distinct disorders based on the site of infection. Oral herpes,(HSV-1) the visible symptoms of which are colloquially called cold sores or fever blisters, is an infection of the face or mouth. Genital herpes, (HSV-2) known simply as herpes, is the second most common form of herpes.

Signs and symptoms: HSV infection causes several distinct medical disorders. Common infection of the skin or mucosa may affect the face and mouth (orofacial herpes), genitalia (genital herpes), or hands (herpetic whitlow). More serious disorders occur when the virus infects and damages the eye (herpes keratitis), or invades the central nervous system, damaging the brain (herpes encephalitis).

Patients with immature or suppressed immune systems, such as newborns, transplant recipients, or AIDS patients are prone to severe complications from HSV infections. HSV infection has also been associated with cognitive deficits of bipolar disorder, and Alzheimer's disease, although this is often dependent on the genetics of the infected person. In all cases HSV is never removed from the body by the immune system. (Note: herpes zoster, the chicken pox virus also stays in the body and is the cause of shingles).

Following a primary infection, the virus enters the nerves at the site of primary infection, migrates to the cell body of the neuron, and becomes latent in the ganglion. As a result of primary infection, the body produces antibodies to the particular type of HSV involved, preventing a subsequent infection of that type at a different site. In HSV-1 infected individuals, sero-conversion after an oral infection will prevent additional HSV-1 infections such as whitlow, some genital herpes, and herpes of the eye. Prior HSV-1 sero-conversion seems to reduce the symptoms of a later HSV-2 infection, although HSV-2 can still be contracted. Many people infected with HSV-2 display no physical symptoms—individuals with no symptoms are described as asymptomatic or as having <u>subclinical herpes</u>.

Alzheimer's disease: HSV-1 has been proposed as a possible cause of Alzheimer's disease. In the presence of a certain gene variation (APOE-epsilon4 allele carriers), HSV-1 appears to be particularly damaging to the nervous system and increases one's risk of developing Alzheimer's disease. The virus interacts with the components and receptors of lipoproteins, which may lead to the development of Alzheimer's disease. Herpes simplex virus type 1 DNA is localized within the <u>beta-amyloid plaques</u> that characterize Alzheimer's disease. It suggests that this virus is a major cause of the plaques and, hence, probably a significant etiological factor in Alzheimer's disease.

Causes: Herpes Simplex is contracted through direct contact with an active lesion or body fluid of an infected person. Herpes transmission occurs between discordant partners: a person with a history of infection (HSV sero-positive) can pass the virus to an HSV sero-negative person. Herpes simplex virus 2 is typically contracted through direct skin-to-skin contact with an infected individual but can also be contacted via exposure to infected saliva, semen, vaginal fluid or the fluid from herpetic blisters. To infect a new individual, HSV travels through tiny breaks in the skin or mucous membranes in the mouth or genital areas. Even microscopic abrasions on mucous membranes are sufficient to allow viral entry. HSV asymptomatic shedding occurs at some time in most individuals infected with herpes. It can occur more than a week before or after a symptomatic recurrence in 50% of cases. Virus enters into susceptible cells via entry receptors.

Infected people that show no visible symptoms may still shed and transmit virus through their skin: asymptomatic shedding may represent the most common form of HSV-2 transmission. Asymptomatic shedding is more frequent within the first 12 months of acquiring HSV. Concurrent infection with HIV increases the frequency and duration of asymptomatic shedding.

There are indications that some individuals may have much lower patterns of shedding, but evidence supporting this is not fully verified: no significant differences are seen in the frequency of asymptomatic shedding when comparing persons with one to twelve annual recurrences to those with no recurrences. Antibodies that develop following an initial infection with a type of HSV prevents re-infection with the same virus type.

Note:—a person with a history of orofacial infection caused by HSV-1 cannot contract herpes whitlow or a genital infection caused by HSV-1. In a monogamous couple, a sero-negative female runs a greater than 30% per year risk of contracting an HSV infection from a sero-positive male partner. If an oral HSV-1 infection is contracted first, sero-conversion will have occurred after 6 weeks to provide protective antibodies against a future genital HSV-1 infection.

Nutritional factors: Herpes is a virus that many people carry in their bodies without knowing it. The herpes simplex virus can lie dormant in your body for years, and an outbreak of cold sores may suddenly occur. The herpes virus causes cold sores, chicken pox, genital herpes and shingles. Though medications are commonly used to suppress and treat herpes, the attacks can also be controlled through the diet.

Avoiding certain types of foods can reduce the number of herpes outbreaks that you experience. Avoid wheat products like wheat germ, wheat bread and cream of wheat are another major culprit for triggering herpes outbreaks. While they are generally healthy as they provide vitamins and minerals, the arginine content in

139

wheat products is of particular concern to carriers of the herpes simplex virus. Wheat germ, especially, has 1,330mg of herpes-activating arginine in each serving.

Peanuts may trigger herpes outbreaks, so you should limit your consumption of them if you have the herpes simplex virus. Foods high in the amino acid arginine speed up cell replication and may cause the herpes virus to become more active. The amino acid lysine works good and is in opposition to arginine, decreasing herpes outbreaks.

The higher the lysine-to-arginine ratio of a food is, the lower the likelihood it has to cause a herpes outbreak. Peanuts have 144mg of lysine but also 1,450mg of arginine per serving. This gives them a low lysine-to-arginine ratio of 0.28. Sesame seeds are another food that may trigger outbreaks of herpes. There are 150mg lysine in a serving of sesame seeds and 1,240mg arginine. The lysine-to-arginine ratio of sesame seeds is 0.25. Grape Juice is also high in arginine and is likely to cause herpes outbreaks. Instead of drinking grape juice, a person with the herpes virus should **drink vegetable juice or milk, which is lower in arginine**. Avoid nuts and seeds if you are prone to having herpes outbreaks, in favor of foods like cheese and beef, which are high in lysine.

Treatment: There is no method to eradicate herpes virus from the body, but antiviral medications can reduce the frequency, duration, and severity of outbreaks. Analgesics such as ibuprofen and acetaminophen can reduce pain and fever. Topical anesthetic treatments such as prilocaine, lidocaine, benzocaine or tetracaine can also relieve itching and pain.

Anti-virals: There are several antivirals that are effective for treating herpes including: acyclovir (acyclovir), valacyclovir (valacyclovir), famcyclovir, and pencyclovir. Acyclovir was the first discovered and is now available in generic. Valacyclovir is also available as a generic. Evidence supports the use of acyclovir and valacyclovir in the treatment of herpes labialis as well as herpes infections in people with cancer. The evidence to support the use of acyclovir in primary herpetic gingivostomatitis is less strong. Topical anti-virals: A number of topical anti-virals are effective for herpes labialis including acyclovir, pencyclovir, and docosanol.

Alternative medicine: There are a number of small studies showing possible benefit from L-lysine, aspirin, lemon balm, Echinacea, zinc, topical zinc, licorice root cream and/or aloe vera in treatment.

Summary: Herpes simplex is divided into two types: HSV 1 and HSV 2. HSV 1 causes primarily mouth, throat, face, eye, and central nervous system infections, whereas HSV 2 causes primarily anogenital infections. However, each may cause infections in all areas.

HIGH BLOOD PRESSURE (HYPERTENSION): Hypertension (HTN) or High Blood Pressure (HBP) is sometimes called "Arterial Hypertension". It is a chronic medical condition in which the blood pressure in the arteries is elevated. This requires the heart to work harder than normal to circulate blood through the blood vessels.

Blood pressure involves two measurements, systolic and diastolic, which depend on whether the heart muscle is contracting (systole) or relaxed between beats (diastole). Normal blood pressure at rest is within the range of 100-140mmHg systolic (top reading) and 60-90mmHg diastolic (bottom reading). High blood pressure is said to be present if it is persistently at or above 140/90 mmHg.

Hypertension is classified as either primary (essential) hypertension or secondary hypertension. Primary hypertension means high blood pressure with no obvious underlying medical cause. Secondary hypertension is caused by other conditions that affect the kidneys, arteries, heart or endocrine system. Hypertension is a major risk factor for stroke, myocardial infarction (heart attacks), heart failure, aneurysms of the arteries (e.g. aortic aneurysm), peripheral arterial disease and is a cause of chronic kidney disease. Even moderate elevation of arterial blood pressure is associated with a shortened life expectancy.

Signs and symptoms: A proportion of people with high blood pressure reports headaches (particularly at the back of the head and in the morning), as well as lightheadedness, vertigo, (dizziness) tinnitus (buzzing or hissing in the ears), altered vision or fainting episodes. These symptoms however are more likely to be related more to anxiety than the high blood pressure. Some additional signs and symptoms may suggest secondary hypertension, i.e. hypertension due to an identifiable cause such as kidney diseases or endocrine diseases.

For example, truncal obesity, glucose intolerance, moon facies, a "buffalo hump" and purple striae suggest Cushing's syndrome. Also, Thyroid disease can also cause hypertension and have characteristic symptoms and signs. An abdominal bruit may be an indicator of renal artery stenosis (a narrowing of the arteries supplying the kidneys), while decreased blood pressure in the lower extremities with absent or delayed absent femoral arterial pulses may indicate aortic coarctation which is a narrowing of the aorta shortly after it leaves the heart.

Hypertensive crises = Hypertensive emergency: Severely elevated blood pressure (equal to or greater than a systolic 180 or diastolic of 110 — sometime termed malignant or accelerated hypertension) is referred to as a "hypertensive crisis", as blood pressures above these levels are known to increase the risk of complications. People with blood pressures in this range are more likely to report headaches and dizziness than the general population.

Visual deterioration or breathlessness due to heart failure or a general feeling of malaise due to renal failure are other symptoms accompanying a hypertensive crisis. Most people with a hypertensive crisis are known to have elevated blood pressure, but additional triggers may have led to a sudden rise. A "hypertensive emergency" is diagnosed when there is evidence of direct damage to one or more organs as a result of the severely elevated blood pressure. This may include hypertensive encephalopathy, caused by brain swelling and dysfunction, and characterized by headaches and an altered level of consciousness (confusion or drowsiness).

 Retinal papilloedema and/or fundal hemorrhages and exudates are another sign of target organ damage. Chest pain may indicate heart muscle damage (which may progress to myocardial infarction) or sometimes aortic dissection, the tearing of the inner wall of the aorta. Breathlessness, cough, and the expectoration of blood-stained sputum are characteristic signs of pulmonary edema, (the swelling of lung tissue due to left ventricular failure or an inability of the left ventricle of the heart to adequately pump blood from the lungs into the arterial system).

Rapid deterioration of kidney function (acute kidney injury) and microangiopathic hemolytic anemia (destruction of blood cells) may also occur. Use of oral medications to lower the BP gradually over 24 to 48 hours is advocated in hypertensive emergencies. However, hypertension is rarely accompanied by any symptoms, and its identification is usually through screening, or when seeking healthcare for an unrelated problem.

Nutritional Factors that aid in reducing or controlling hypertension: Dietary and lifestyle changes can improve blood pressure control and decrease the risk of associated health complications, although drug treatment is often necessary in people for whom lifestyle changes prove ineffective or insufficient.

Skim Milk. Drinking heart-healthy skim milk or 1 percent milk will provide you with calcium and vitamin D: these nutrients work to help reduce blood pressure.

Spinach. A green leafy delight, spinach is low in calories, high in fiber, and packed with heart-healthy nutrients like potassium, folate, and magnesium: key ingredients for lowering and maintaining blood pressure level.

Unsalted Sunflower seeds are also a great source of magnesium. A nutritious snack, but be sure to buy them unsalted since salted sunflower seeds are high in sodium, which you want to avoid. Avoid sodium is a good rule to follow in most cases.

Beans. Nutritious and versatile, beans (including black, white, navy, lima, pinto, and kidney) are chock-full of soluble fiber, magnesium and potassium, all excellent ingredients for lowering blood pressure and improving overall heart health

Baked White Potato. Potatoes are rich in both magnesium and potassium, two vital nutrients for heart health. When potassium is low, the body retains extra sodium (and too much sodium raises blood pressure). On the other hand, when you eat a potassium-rich diet, the body becomes more efficient at getting rid of excess sodium. Like potassium, magnesium is also a key player in promoting healthy blood flow. Therefore, maintaining a healthy balance of both minerals (potassium and magnesiumcan help keep high blood pressure at bay.

Bananas. This functional fruit is packed with potassium and magnesium, so it's a great choice for an on-the-go snack that will lower blood pressure and improve heart health.

Soybeans. Soybeans are another excellent source of potassium and magnesium. Look for soybeans in the pod (edamame) in the freezer case at your grocery store: for a healthy snack, boil one cup and pop them directly out of the shell into your mouth.

Dark Chocolate. Eating about 30 calories a day of dark chocolate: just one tiny square was shown to help lower blood pressure. Choose dark chocolate consisting of at least 70 percent cocoa powder or greater.

HIVES: Hives, which is medically called urticaria, is not contagious. Hives is a skin disorder that results in red, sometimes itching patches of raised skin. Hives are an allergic reaction to something you have come into contact with at one point or another. You could have touched a new plant, used a new detergent or soap, even medications you are taking can cause hives. They can also be caused by too much stress in your life - this is known as stress hives.

Since no two people have the same reaction to an allergen, hives are not contagious: hives are a personal allergic reaction. Even if you walked around rubbing your allergen onto someone else who is not allergic to it, they may not get hives even if you do. Hives occur when your body thinks something is there that it does not agree with, called an allergen.

The immune system then releases what are called histamines into the blood stream to attack the allergen and make it go away. In turn, to let you know there is a problem, your body breaks out in these small red and itchy sometimes burning bumps or raised areas: you can even get hives on face.

The only way you could get hives from someone else is if they had your allergen in their hand and rubbed it on you. For example, if you were allergic to a specific soap, another person would have to rub that soap on you for you to get hives. But you still did not catch hives from that person, you got them from the soap. You can still use the same wash cloths or towels, or sit on the same toilet seat as someone who has hives.

Signs and symptoms: Red, flat or slightly raised patches of skin can be small or large, and generally appear quite fast and disappear on their own within hours or days. Hives can be as small as a few millimeters and as large as inches, and can even join together (coalesce) to become large areas called plaques. Hives that join together all over your body are generally known as body hives. These are quite itchy in nature and can burn.

Since hives can occur due to medications, exercise, overexertion, sweating (heat hives), foods and many other things, sometimes there is no known cause for certain cases. You may undergo extreme amounts of testing and still not know what caused your hives. But you can be certain that you cannot give it to your friends, family or pets by being around them or touching them. Hives can occur on any part of the body including your tongue, ears, lips or face (known as facial hives). Interesting: the only areas that cases have not been seen on are the palms of the hands and the soles of the feet. Hives can move from one area to another within minutes, and can disappear and reappear within hours.

Nutritional Factors: It is notable that most allergic symptoms worsen after the consumption of foods such as eggs, shellfish, fish, strawberries, pineapple, tomatoes, chocolate, alcohol (especially wine and beer) or smoking. There are other foods that contain great amounts of histamine, or release histamine. During the allergies, the body reacts to them by producing extra histamine, hence anti-histamines drugs are recommended. It must be noted that each individual has different tolerance level for histamine thus different people will react differently on different histamine levels.

If your histamine tolerance level is reached: it overflows causing allergic symptoms happen. The fermenting of foods lead to histamine is production as in cheese, grits, vinegar and alcoholic drinks. Unfortunately some foods have natural extra amounts of histamine as tomato, eggplant and spinach. Food additives including azo dyes, tartrazine and preservatives trigger the histamine releasing. Benzoates which occur naturally in some foods also cause histamine to be released hence making them to be listed as those that need to be avoided so as to reduce the allergic symptoms.

Others food that should be avoided. Fish and eggs should be avoided. Most of these products will produce high levels of histamine that cause a histamine food poisoning, especially fish, shellfish, anchovies and sardines if they start going bad. Avoid all processed, smoked or fermented meats as sandwich meat, sausage, wiener, bologna, salami, pepperoni, smoked ham, bacon. Leftovers are easily acted upon by bacteria hence histamine is produced especially in protein based leftover kept at room or refrigerator temperatures. To avoid this production of histamines, freeze all the leftovers to stop histamine production.

Avoid all fermented milk products such as cheeses, yogurt, buttermilk, and kefir, sour cream. Fruits to avoid are oranges, grapefruit, lemon, lime, cherries, grapes, apricots, avocados, raspberries, cranberries, prunes, loganberries, dates, raisins, currants-fresh or dried. In addition bananas, papayas, pineapple, and strawberries also release histamine. Vegetables to avoid are tomatoes and their products like tomato sauces, catsup and others, soy products, spinach, red beans, eggplant, pumpkin.

All vegetables packed in vinegar or salt as olives, pickles, relish and other fermented vegetables as sauerkraut must be avoided. All types of alcohol must be avoided: including beer and wine for they can cause histamines to be released. Other foods to be avoided in controlling and treating hives are some food addictives and food colors, seasons such as cinnamon, cloves, vinegar, chili, anise, nutmeg, soy sauce and curry powder, beverages such as, coffee, chocolate, cocoa, cola, alcohol and any others that will cause allergy in you. <u>Taking one glass of lemon water at least 8 times a day is recommended.</u>

HYPOGLYCEMIA: Hypoglycemia (low blood sugar) is not a disease but rather a sign of low blood sugar. In actuality, while some or many of the symptoms of hypoglycemia may be present, it is rarely confirmed or documented. The presence of true, documented hypoglycemia in the absence of diabetes treatment must be evaluated comprehensively by an endocrinologist.

 Hypoglycemia most often affects those at the extremes of age, such as infants and the elderly, but may happen at any age. Hypoglycemia is generally defined as a serum glucose level (the amount of sugar or glucose in your blood) below 70 mg/dL.

As a medical problem, hypoglycemia is diagnosed by the presence of three key features (known as Whipple's triad). <u>Whipple's triad</u> consists of: <u>*symptoms consistent with hypoglycemia</u>, <u>*a low plasma glucose concentration and or high plasma insulin</u>, and <u>*relief of symptoms after the plasma glucose level is raised</u>. The body regulates its glucose level by the actions of different hormones. These hormones include insulin (which lowers the blood sugar level) and other hormones that raise blood sugar (such as glucagon, epinephrine, growth hormone). Both insulin and glucagon are manufactured in the pancreas, an organ near the stomach which assists the digestive tract. Special cells in the pancreas, called beta cells, make insulin. Alpha cells in the pancreas make glucagon.   The role of insulin is to help in the absorption of glucose from the blood by causing it to be stored in the liver or be transported into other tissues of the body (i.e., fat cells) for storage).

Glucagon increases the amount of glucose in the blood by breaking down stored triglycerides (body fat) and glycogen to glucose and releasing this glucose into the bloodstream. <u>Insulin and glucagon</u>

are usually correctly balanced if the liver and pancreas are functioning normally.

Epinephrine (adrenalin), a stress hormone, is made in the adrenal gland and in certain cells in the central nervous system. Epinephrine also elevates blood glucose levels by making glucose available for the body during a time of stress. Other hormones also help in raising the level of blood glucose, like cortisol made by the adrenal gland and growth hormone made by the pituitary gland. When these mechanism are not working properly, hypoglycemia can result.

Signs and Symptoms of hypoglycemia typically appear at levels below 70 mg/dL. Some people may feel symptoms above this level. Levels below 50 mg/dL affect brain function, i.e., altered mental status or unconsciousness. Your body needs a steady supply of sugar (glucose) in order to function properly.

If glucose levels become too low, as occurs with hypoglycemia, it can have these effects on your brain: Confusion, abnormal behavior or both, such as the inability to complete routine tasks. Visual disturbances, such as double vision and blurred vision, Seizures, though uncommon, Loss of consciousness, though uncommon.

Hypoglycemia may also cause other signs and symptoms: Heart palpitations, Shakiness, Anxiety, Sweating, Hunger, Tingling sensation around the mouth. These signs and symptoms aren't specific to hypoglycemia. There may be other causes. A blood sample to test your blood sugar (glucose) at the time of these signs and symptoms is the only way to know for sure that hypoglycemia is the cause.

Causes: Common causes of low blood sugar include the following:

- Overmedication with insulin or antidiabetic pills (for example, sulfonylurea drugs such as Diabeta, Glyburide, Glipizide, Micronase, etc.)
- Use of medications such as beta blockers, pentamidine, and sulfamethoxazole and trimethoprim (Bactrim, Septra)
- Use of alcohol
- Missed meals
- Reactive hypoglycemia is the result of the delayed insulin release after a meal has been absorbed and occurs 4-6 hours after eating.
- Severe infection
- Cancer causing poor oral intake or cancer involving the liver
- Adrenal insufficiency
- Kidney failure and/or Liver failure
- Congenital, genetic defects in the regulation of insulin release (congenital hyperinsulinism)
- Congenital conditions associated with increased insulin release (infant born to a diabetic mother, birth trauma, reduced oxygen delivery during birth, major birth stress, Beckwith-Wiedemann syndrome, and rarer genetic conditions)
- Insulinoma or insulin-producing tumor
- Other tumors like hepatoma, mesothelioma, and fibrosarcoma

Most cases of hypoglycemia in adults happen in people with diabetes mellitus. Diabetes has two forms, type 1 (loss of all insulin production) and type 2 (inadequate insulin production due to resistance to the actions of insulin). People with type 1 diabetes must take insulin to control their glucose level: if they skip a meal or have a decreased appetite without changing their insulin dose, they may develop hypoglycemia.

Insulin is also used to treat some people with type 2 diabetes. If a person with type 1 diabetes accidentally takes too much insulin, or a person with type 2 diabetes accidentally takes too much of their oral medications or insulin, he or she may develop hypoglycemia. Even when a diabetic patient takes medications correctly, improper meals, odd mealtimes, or excessive exercise may result in hypoglycemia.

Nutritional factors: There is no hard and fast rule to be followed while making your diet plan if you are suffering from hypoglycemia. It is just that you have to have your food at scheduled times to avoid getting faint all of a sudden. It is the same normal food stuff you should have, but in a different way than the normal. Don't panic.

The following are some tips to help you set up your own diet plan.

- Break down your daily amount of intake into nothing less than 6 meals a day.
- Try to include as much high fiber, complex carbohydrates, as well as protein and good fats in your diet.
- Try eating, whole grain, fresh fruits and green vegetables
- Cut down on your sugar intake.
- Have sweets but as a part of your total meal and only at special meals: and that too in small quantity
- Stay away from food stuff containing of caffeine such as coffee, chocolates , colas and tea.
- Never have alcohol on an empty stomach and try to reduce the intake of alcohol.
- Watch your weight, if that happens to be a concern.
- Exercise daily if that is possible for you.

Reactive hypoglycemia is a chronic condition which calls for special treatment. With a good and a well planned diet program, you can definitely expect a steady progress to healthy living.

Some healthy snack choices could be as follows:

- Fruits combine with two whole grain crackers.
- One half peanut sandwiches on bread with raw carrots.
- Low fat cheese placed between two whole grain crackers.
- Simple and plain yogurt mixed along with fresh fruits.
- Low fat milk with banana can also be a good choice for snack.
- Apple with cheese on a half sliced whole wheat bread. Divide your meals this way: Breakfast, Snack, Lunch, Snack, Dinner, Snack. That actually makes 6 meals for the entire day.

IMMUNE SYSTEM DEPRESSION: The immune system is responsible for protecting your body from things that could do it harm. It is composed of external features, such as skin, and internal features, such as the inflammatory response to bacteria, viruses and chemicals as well the inflammatory response to cancers. It is very important to keep our immune systems in tip-top shape.

Signs and Symptoms: A healthy, functioning immune system results in symptoms such as: weight loss, bodily pain, stress fatigue and even fever. Only when the immune system is not functioning correctly does it get out of control and cause major medical problems. For example, if we are infected by the flu virus we often experience symptoms such as fever, chills, aches and pains.

Fever is evidence of the body's immune system is working: it is actually fighting the infective agent (the bacteria or virus): and this can be a good thing. Also, it is possible for the body to produce too few stress hormones "stress fatigue". This inhibits the body's immune system from turning off when it is not needed. This, malfunction of the brain, tells the immune system to keep on fighting when there is nothing to fight, other than the body itself. This can leads to the chronic fatigue syndrome. This can also result in disorders of the immune system, such as lupus and rheumatoid arthritis.

Causes: Stress depress the immune system. Stress can take the form of depression, anxiety or panic. Stress may also take the form of fatigue due to lack of sleep and prolonged physical exertion. When you are chronically stressed, your brain signals the body to produce stress hormones. These hormones soak the immune system, which impairs its ability to fight foreign substances or chemicals that can be harmful to the body.

People whose immune systems are consistently under stress are unable to respond to illness quickly and are more susceptible to contracting viral and bacterial infections as well as depression and anxiety disorders. Sugar depresses the immune system. Vitamin C is needed by white blood cells. These white blood cells phagocytize (gobble up) viruses and bacteria.

White blood cells require a 50 times higher concentration of vitamin "C" inside the cell as outside so they have to accumulate vitamin C. There is something called a "phagocytic index" which tells you how rapidly particular white blood cells (macrophage or lymphocyte) can gobble up a virus, bacteria, and/or cancer cells.

It was in the 1970's that Linus Pauling realized that white blood cells need a high dose of vitamin "C" and that is when he came up with his theory that you need high doses of vitamin C to combat the common cold. It is now known that glucose and vitamin C have similar chemical structures, so when the sugar levels go up in the blood stream, they compete with vitamin "C" for entrance into the white blood cell. And the thing that mediates the entry of glucose into the cells is the same thing that mediates the entry of vitamin C into the cells. If there is more glucose around than vitamin "C", there is going to be less vitamin C allowed into the cell. It doesn't take much: a blood sugar value of 120 reduces the phagocytic index by 75%.

So when you consume sugar, your immune system slows down to a crawl and this impaired immune system is the root cause of most medical diseases. It doesn't matter what disease we are talking about, whether we are talking about a common cold or about cardiovascular disease, cancer or osteoporosis, the root cause is always going to be at the cellular and molecular level, and more often than not - **sugar** - is going to have their hand in it, if not totally - controlling it. Many health problems, created from ingesting sugar on a habitual basis, are certain.

Simple sugars have been observed to aggravate asthma, move mood swings, trigger personality changes, mental illness and nervous disorders, cause diabetes, and trigger heart disease, gallstones, hypertension, and even arthritis.

Because refined dietary sugars lack minerals, phytonutrients, and vitamins, they must draw upon the body's micro-nutrient stored sources in order to be metabolized or used by the immune system. When these storehouses are depleted, metabolization of cholesterol and fatty acid is impeded, triggers hypertension, heart disease and obesity due to higher concentrations of triglycerides, cholesterol, and thus promoting fatty acid storage around organs and in sub-cutaneous tissue. Because sugar is devoid of phytonutrients, minerals, vitamins, fiber, it has this very deteriorating effect on the immune system. Many researchers agree that <u>sugar consumption in America is one of the 3 major causes of most medical diseases, especially age-related, metabolic medical diseases.</u>

Sugar and cancer: Of the over 4 million cancer patients being treated in the U.S. today, almost none are offered any scientifically guided nutrition therapy other than being told to "just eat good foods." Many cancer patients would have a major improvement in their conditions <u>if they controlled and limited the amount of ingested sugar, especially simple carbohydrates made from white flour, sugar and even nonnutritive artificial sweeteners. Glucose (sugar) is the main substance that fuels cancer.</u>

By slowing the growth of cancer cells, patients <u>make it possible for their immune systems to catch up to the disease</u>. Controlling one's blood-glucose levels through diet, exercise, supplements, meditation and prescription drugs - when necessary - can be <u>one of the most crucial components to a cancer treatment program</u>. The saying "Sugar feeds cancer" is simple. Hence, cancer therapies should attempt to regulate blood-glucose levels through diet, supplements, exercise, medication and stress reduction. Since cancer cells derive most of their energy from anaerobic glycolysis, the goal is not to eliminate sugars or carbohydrates entirely from the diet but rather to control blood-glucose within a narrow range to help starve the cancer cells and **boost immune function**.

Nutritional factors: The average American consumes an astounding 2-3 pounds of sugar each week, which is not surprising considering that highly refined sugars in the forms of sucrose (table sugar), dextrose (corn sugar), and high-fructose corn syrup are being processed into so many foods such as bread, breakfast cereal, peanut butter, mayonnaise, ketchup, spaghetti sauce, and a plethora of microwave meals. In the last 20 years, we have increased sugar consumption in the U.S. from 26 pounds to 135 lbs. of sugar per person per year! Prior to the turn of this century (1887-1890), the average consumption was only 5 lbs. per person per year! Cardiovascular disease, Neuro-psych metabolic diseases (depression and Alzheimer) and cancer was virtually unknown in the early 1900's.

The "glycemic index" is a measure of how a given food affects blood-glucose levels, with each food being assigned a numbered rating. The lower the rating, the slower the absorption and digestion process, which provides a more gradual, healthier infusion of sugars into the bloodstream. On the other hand, a high rating means that blood-glucose levels are increased quickly, which stimulates the pancreas to secrete insulin to drop blood-sugar levels quickly. These rapid fluctuations of blood-sugar levels are not healthy because of the stress they place on the body.

One of sugar's major drawbacks is that it raises the insulin level, which then inhibits the release of growth hormone, thyroid hormone and glucagon, which in turn depresses the immune system as well as triggers depression, anxiety disorders and more complicated neurological diseases and promotes obesity, cholesterol and triglyceride problems such as heart disease, hypertension and diabetes, etc.

INSOMNIA / SLEEP DEPRIVATION: Insomnia is defined as difficulty initiating or maintaining sleep, or both, despite adequate opportunity and time to sleep, leading to impaired daytime functioning. Insomnia is very common and occurs in 30% to 50% of the general population. Insomnia affects people of all ages, although it is more common in adults and its frequency increases with age. In general, women are affected more frequently than men.

 Insomnia can also be classified based on the underlying reasons for insomnia such as sleep hygiene, medical conditions, sleep disorders, stress factors, etc. It is important to make a distinction between insomnia and other similar terminology: short duration sleep and sleep deprivation. Short duration sleep may be normal in some individuals who may require less time for sleep without feeling daytime impairment, the central symptom in the definition of insomnia. In insomnia, adequate time and opportunity for sleep is available, whereas in sleep deprivation, lack of sleep is due to lack of opportunity or time to sleep because of voluntary or intentional avoidance of sleep.

Signs and Symptoms and Causes: Insomnia may be due to poor quality or quantity of sleep. Insomnia may have many causes and, as described earlier, it can be classified based upon the underlying cause. Situational and stress factors leading to insomnia may include: jet lag, physical discomfort (hot, cold, lighting, noise, unfamiliar surroundings), working different shifts, stressful life situations (divorce or separation, death of a loved one, losing a job, preparing for an examination), illicit drug use, cigarette smoking, caffeine intake prior to going to bed, alcohol intoxication or withdrawal, or certain medications. Most of these factors may be short-term and transient, and therefore insomnia may resolve when the underlying factor is removed or corrected. Sleep hygiene can play an important role in insomnia. Poor sleep hygiene includes physical factors such as: using the bedroom for things other than sleeping, eating or exercising prior to sleep, going to bed hungry, sleeping in a room with too much noise or lighting, or doing work in bed.

Medical and psychiatric conditions may also contribute to insomnia. Some of these common medical conditions may include:

breathing problems from chronic heart or lung disease (asthma, chronic obstructive pulmonary disease (COPD), congestive heart failure, obstructive sleep apnea), obesity, acid reflux, hyperthyroidism, urinary problems (frequent urination, urinary incontinence), chronic pain, fibromyalgia, Parkinson's disease, or dementia. Common psychiatric problems can be responsible for insomnia including: depression, psychosis, mania, anxiety, or post-traumatic stress disorder (PTSD).

Some common physiologic conditions can lead to insomnia such as: menopause, menstrual cycle, pregnancy, fever, or pain. Other causes of insomnia may be related to sleep disorders including: sleep walking, sleep apnea, restless leg syndrome (RLS creeping sensations in the leg during sleep, relieved by leg movement), periodic limb movement disorder (involuntary repeated leg movement during sleep), or circadian sleep disturbance (unusual sleep time due to disturbed biological clock).

Nutritional factors: Many healthy foods contain ingredients that can act as sedatives or boost certain hormones to induce sleep. By altering your diet, particularly the foods you eat right in the hours before bedtime, these natural cures for insomnia will have you sleeping peacefully. Opt for items that are calcium-rich when you're trying to choose foods to cure insomnia.

By drinking an eight-ounce glass of low fat milk a few hours before you go to bed, for example, you can increase serotonin levels in your system, naturally, to help you get a sound night of sleep. Other foods in this group that cure insomnia include yogurt, and cheeses. If you can't eat dairy, consider curing sleeplessness with items like tofu, salmon or calcium-fortified orange juice and fortified cereal with almond milk.

Eat foods that reduce stress levels, i.e. less caffeine. Remember, stress can lead to sleeplessness. Choose foods high in magnesium to cure insomnia like <u>nuts</u> (particularly <u>cashews</u>, <u>pine nuts</u> and <u>almonds</u>), <u>oat bran, artichokes, spinach and black beans</u>. <u>These magnesium rich foods</u> also help <u>combat the anxiety</u> that keeps you awake at night. Add <u>bananas</u> to your diet to serve as natural remedies for insomnia. Bananas have a high level of magnesium and <u>vitamin B6</u> that can also <u>help generate serotonin</u> to keep your internal clock functioning properly to both prevent fatigue during the day and help you fall asleep at night.

Other foods that fit into this insomnia cure include <u>bell peppers, tuna, chicken, turkey, spinach and halibut</u> <u>within five hours of bedtime has been shown to be a treatment for insomnia by having a sedative effect</u>. Consider items with a high glycemic index when you choose foods to cure insomnia. *Because of their affect on blood glucose and insulin levels, however, this insomnia cure should be used with caution if you have a medical condition like diabetes or are trying to reduce carbs to lose weight.*

Summary: The following is a list of foods known to help induce sleep. Calcium rich foods such as: Low fat milk, yogurt, cheese, calcium fortified almond milk, calcium-fortified orange juice, salmon. Magnesium rich foods such as: bananas, nuts, (i.e., cashews, almonds, pine nuts, pecans), oat bran, oatmeal products, artichokes, spinach and black beans. Other foods that fit into the insomnia cure include: bell peppers, tuna, chicken, turkey, and halibut all within five hours of bedtime. Also, reduce caffeine products.

IRRITABLE BOWEL SYNDROME: Irritable bowel syndrome (IBS), or Spastic Colon is a symptom-based diagnosis characterized by chronic abdominal pain, discomfort, bloating, and alteration of bowel habits. <u>As a functional bowel disorder, IBS has no known organic cause</u>. Historically a diagnosis of exclusion, a diagnosis of IBS can now be made on the basis of symptoms alone, in the absence of alarm features such as age of onset greater than 50 years, weight loss, hematochezia, systemic signs of infection or colitis, or family history of inflammatory bowel disease.

Several conditions may present as IBS including celiac disease, fructose malabsorption, mild infections, parasitic infections like giardiasis, several inflammatory bowel diseases, bile acid malabsorption, functional chronic constipation, and chronic functional abdominal pain. In IBS, routine clinical tests yield no abnormalities. The exact cause of IBS is unknown.

The most common theory is that IBS is a disorder of the interaction between the brain and the gastrointestinal tract, although there may also be abnormalities in the gut flora or the immune system. IBS is a source of chronic pain, fatigue, and other symptoms and contributes to work absenteeism. The high prevalence of IBS and significant effects on quality of life make IBS a disease with a high social cost. IBS can be classified as either diarrhea-predominant (IBS-D), constipation-predominant (IBS-C) or IBS with alternating stool pattern or pain-predominant (IBS-A).

Signs and Symptoms: diarrhea and/or constipation and pain are classic symptoms. Onset of IBS is more likely to occur after an infection (post-infectious IBS), a stressful life event, or after onset of maturity. The primary symptoms of IBS are abdominal pain or discomfort in association with frequent diarrhea or constipation, and a change in bowel habits. There may also be urgency for bowel movements, a feeling of incomplete evacuation (tenesmus), bloating or abdominal distention. In some cases, the symptoms are relieved by bowel movements. People with IBS, more commonly than others, have gastro-esophageal reflux (GERD), symptoms relating to the genitourinary system, chronic fatigue syndrome, fibromyalgia, headache, backache, depression and anxiety.

Causes: The cause of IBS is unknown, but several hypotheses have been proposed. The risk of developing IBS increases six-fold after acute gastrointestinal infection. Further risk factors are young age, prolonged fever, anxiety, and depression. "Psychological factors" may be important in the etiology of IBS.

Nutritional factors and Treatments: Although there is no cure for IBS, there are treatments that attempt to relieve symptoms, including dietary adjustments, medication and psychological interventions. A number of treatments have been found to be better than placebo, including: fiber, peppermint oil and antispasmodics. Diet: Some people with IBS are likely to have food intolerances. Many different dietary modifications have been attempted to improve the symptoms of IBS. Some are effective in certain sub-populations.

As lactose intolerance and IBS have such similar symptoms a trial of a lactose-free diet is often recommended. A diet restricting fructose intake has been shown to successfully treat the symptoms in a dose-dependent manner in patients with fructose malabsorption and IBS. However, the very act of eating or drinking can provoke an overreaction of the gastro-colic response in some patients with IBS due to their heightened visceral sensitivity.

Fiber: There is convincing evidence that soluble fiber supplementation (e.g., psyllium) is effective in the general IBS population. It acts as a bulking agent, and for many IBS-D patients, it allows for a more consistent stool. For IBS-C patients, it seems to allow for a softer, moister, more easily passable stool.

Insoluble fiber (e.g., bran) has not been found to be effective for IBS. In some people, insoluble fiber supplementation may aggravate symptoms. **Medications** may consist of stool softeners and laxatives in constipation-predominant IBS, and antidiarrheals (e.g., opiate, opioid, or opioid analogs such as loperamide, levsin, diphenoxylate) in diarrhea-predominant IBS for mild symptoms and stronger opiates such as codeine, morphine and oxycodone for severe cases. Drugs affecting serotonin (5-HT) in the intestines can help reduce symptoms.

 Serotonin stimulates the gut motility and so agonists (like serotonin) can help constipation-predominate irritable bowel, while antagonists (opposite serotonin) can help diarrhea-predominant irritable bowel. **Laxatives**: For patients who do not adequately respond to dietary fiber, osmotic laxatives such as polyethylene glycol, sorbitol, and lactulose can help avoid "cathartic colon" which has been associated with stimulant laxatives.

Among the osmotic laxatives, 17–26 grams/day of polyethylene glycol (PEG) has been well studied. Lubiprostone (Amitiza), is a gastrointestinal agent used for the treatment of constipation-predominant IBS. It is well tolerated in adults, including elderly patients. Lubiprostone acts by producing a chloride-rich fluid secretion. These secretions soften the stool, increase motility, and promote spontaneous bowel movements. Unlike many laxative products, Lubiprostone does not show signs of tolerance, dependency, or altered serum electrolyte concentration.

Antispasmodics for diarrhea and cramping. There are three classes of antispasmodics, or drugs that decrease gut contraction and spasm: Anticholinergics work by blocking the parasympathetic branch of the autonomic nervous system [e.g., dicyclomine (Bentyl), hyoscyamine (Anaspaz, Levsin), Donnatal. (Donnatal combines two anticholinergic drugs called atropine and scopolamine with a barbiturate antianxiety drug called Phenobarbital)]. Direct smooth muscle relaxants act directly upon the smooth muscle of the gut and may be the most effective of the antispasmodics, but these drugs are not available in the United States. Peppermint oil is thought to work by decreasing calcium entry into muscle cells, resulting in muscle relaxation. Enteric-coated preparations may be preferable to unprotected peppermint because they allow delivery of the peppermint oil to the colon. The use of antispasmodic drugs [e.g., anticholinergics such as hyoscyamine, (Levsin) or dicyclomine] may help patients, especially those with cramps or diarrhea.

Tricyclic antidepressants: Elavil, there is strong evidence that low doses of tricyclic antidepressants can be effective for irritable bowel syndrome. **Other agents: Magnesium aluminum silicates** can be effective for IBS, abdominal bloating and flatulence, giving more credibility to the potential role of bacterial overgrowth in some patients with IBS.

Domperidone, a dopamine receptor blocker and a para-sympathomimetic, has been shown to reduce bloating and abdominal pain: defecation was similarly improved. **Opioids**: the use of opioids is controversial due to the potential risk of tolerance, physical dependence and addiction but can be the only relief for some diarrhea predominant cases when other treatment has been ineffective.

Cognitive behavioral therapy: Relaxation therapy has also been found to be helpful. Reducing stress may reduce the frequency and severity of IBS symptoms. Techniques that may be helpful include: Relaxation techniques such as meditation, Physical activities such as yoga or tai chi, Regular exercise such as swimming, walking or running. Exercise helps with IBS. At least 30 minutes of strenuous exercise a day.

Alternative medicine: Due to often unsatisfactory results from medical treatments for IBS up to 50 percent of people turn to complementary alternative medicine. Probiotics can be beneficial in the treatment of IBS, taking 10 billion to 100 billion beneficial bacteria per day is recommended for beneficial results. A number of probiotics have been found to be effective including: Lactobacillus plantarum and Bifidobacteria infantis: however, one review found that only Bifidobacteria infantis showed efficacy.

Some yogurt is made using probiotics that may help ease symptoms of irritable bowel syndrome. Herbal remedies: Peppermint oil (Enteric coated capsules), have been suggested for IBS symptoms in adults and children. **Yoga** may be effective for some with irritable bowel syndrome, especially poses which exercise lower abdominal muscles. Acupuncture may be worth a trial in select patients, but the evidence base for effectiveness is weak. The mind-body or brain-gut interactions has been proposed for irritable bowel syndrome and is gaining increasing research attention.

KIDNEY STONES: A kidney stone, also known as a renal calculus is a solid concretion or crystal aggregation formed in the kidneys from dietary minerals in the urine. Urinary stones are typically classified by their location in the kidney (nephrolithiasis), ureter (ureterolithiasis), or bladder (cystolithiasis), or by their chemical composition (i.e. calcium struvite, or uric acid stones). About 80% of those with kidney stones are men. Men most commonly experience their first episode between 30 and 40 years of age, while for women the age at first presentation is somewhat later. Kidney stones typically leave the body by passage in the urine stream, and many stones are formed and passed without causing symptoms. If stones grow to sufficient size (usually at least 3 millimeters (0.12 in)) they can cause obstruction of the ureter and severe pain.

Signs and symptoms: Ureteral obstruction causes post renal azotemia and hydronephrosis (distension and dilation of the renal pelvis and calyces), as well as spasm of the ureter. This leads to pain, most commonly felt in the flank (the area between the ribs and hip), lower abdomen, and groin (a condition called renal colic).

Renal colic can be associated with nausea, vomiting, fever, blood and/or pus in the urine, and painful urination. Renal colic typically comes in waves lasting 20 to 60 minutes, beginning in the flank or lower back and often radiating to the groin or genitals. The diagnosis of kidney stones is made on the basis of information obtained from the history, physical examination, urinalysis, and radiographic studies. Ultrasound examination and blood tests may also aid in the diagnosis. When a stone causes no symptoms, watchful waiting is a valid option.

For symptomatic stones, pain control is usually the <u>first measure,</u> using medications such as nonsteroidal anti-inflammatory drugs or opioids. More severe cases may require surgical intervention. For example, some stones can be shattered into smaller fragments using **lithotripsy** (i.e., extracorporeal shock wave). Some cases require more invasive forms of surgery.

An example is the percutaneous techniques such as percutaneous nephro-lithotomy. Sometimes, a tube (<u>ureteral stent</u>) may be placed in the ureter to bypass the obstruction and alleviate the symptoms, as well as to prevent ureteral stricture after ureteroscopic stone removal. The hallmark of stones that obstruct the ureter or renal pelvis is <u>excruciating, intermittent pain that radiates from the flank to the groin or to the genital area and inner thigh</u>.

This particular type of pain, known as renal colic, is often described as one of the strongest pain sensations known. Renal colic caused by kidney stones is commonly accompanied by <u>urinary urgency, restlessness, hematuria, sweating, nausea, and vomiting</u>. It typically comes in waves lasting 20 to 60 minutes caused by peristaltic contractions of the ureter as it attempts to expel the stone. The link between the urinary tract, the genital system, and the gastrointestinal tract is the basis of the radiation of pain to the gonads, as well as the nausea and vomiting that are also common in urolithiasis is thought to be genetic in origin. Post renal azotemia and hydronephrosis can be observed following the obstruction of urine flow through one or both ureters.

Causes: <u>Dietary factors</u> that increase the risk of stone formation include <u>low fluid intake </u>and high dietary intake of <u>foods containing animal protein, oxalate compounds</u>, and <u>supplemental calcium</u>. Calcium is one component of the most common type of human kidney stones, (calcium oxalate stones). Some studies suggest people who take supplemental calcium have a higher risk of developing kidney stones. Unlike supplemental calcium, high intakes of dietary calcium do not appear to cause kidney stones and may actually protect against their development. This is perhaps related to the role of calcium in binding ingested oxalate in the gastrointestinal tract. In the urine, oxalate is a very strong promoter of calcium oxalate (stone) precipitation, about 15 times stronger than calcium. For most individuals, however, other risk factors for kidney stones, such as high intakes of dietary oxalates: (i.e., <u>spinach, black tea, rhubarb, chocolate, peanuts, and even strawberries)</u> and <u>low fluid intake</u>, also apple juice, cola drinks: all drinks with high fructose corn syrup probably play a greater role than calcium intake. Other electrolytes appear to influence the formation of kidney stones.

For example, <u>fluoridation of drinking water may increase the risk of kidney stone formation.</u> On the other hand, high intake of dietary <u>potassium, magnesium, calcium, etc., appear to reduce the risk of stone formation</u>. Potassium promotes the urinary excretion of citrate, an inhibitor of urinary crystal formation and dietary magnesium also because like citrate, magnesium is also an inhibitor of urinary crystal formation.

Diets in western nations typically contain more animal protein than the body needs. Urinary excretion of excess sulfurous amino acids (e.g., cysteine and methionine), uric acid and other acidic metabolites from animal protein acidifies the urine. Acidic urine promotes the formation of kidney stones. The body often balances this acidic urinary pH by leaching calcium from the bones, which further promotes the formation of kidney stones.

Low urinary citrate excretion is also commonly found in those with a high dietary intake of animal protein, whereas vegetarians tend to have higher levels of citrate excretion. There is no conclusive data demonstrating a cause-and-effect relationship between alcohol consumption and kidney stones. <u>However, some have theorized that certain behaviors associated with frequent and binge drinking can lead to systemic dehydration, which can in turn lead to the development of kidney stones.</u>

When the urine becomes supersaturated with one or more crystal-forming substances, a seed crystal may form through the process of nucleation. Depending on the chemical composition of the crystal, the stone-forming process may proceed more rapidly when the urine pH is unusually high or low. Supersaturation of the urine with respect to a crystal forming compound is <u>pH-dependent</u>.

 For example, at a pH of 7.0, the solubility of uric acid in urine is 158 mg/100 ml. Reducing the pH to 5.0 decreases the solubility of uric acid to less than 8 mg/100 ml. The formation of uric acid stones requires a combination of hyperuricosuria (high urine uric acid levels) and low urine pH: <u>hyperuricosuria alone is not associated with uric acid stone formation if the urine pH is alkaline (pH above 7.5).</u>

Supersaturation is likely the underlying cause of uric acid and cystine stones, but calcium-based stones (especially calcium oxalate stones) may have a more complex etiology but are definitely associated with foods that contain oxalate. The following are some examples of the most common sources of oxalates, arranged by food group.

It is important to note that the <u>leaves of a plant</u> (spinach, collard greens, black tea, dandelion) almost always contain higher oxalate levels than the roots, stems, and stalks.

<u>Fruits</u>: blackberries, blueberries, raspberries, strawberries, currants, kiwifruit, concord (purple) grapes, figs, tangerines, and plums. <u>Vegetables</u>: spinach, Swiss chard, beet greens, collards, okra, parsley, leeks and quinoa are among the most oxalate-dense vegetables, celery, green beans, rutabagas, and summer squash would be considered moderately dense in oxalates along with nuts, seeds: almonds, cashews, and peanuts. <u>Legumes</u>: soy products, soybeans, tofu. <u>Grains</u>: wheat bran, wheat germ, quinoa (a vegetable often used like a grain). <u>Other</u>: cocoa, chocolate, and black tea.

Nutritional factors: The kidneys play a central role in the urinary system, regulating excretion, the balance of salts in the body and blood pressure. Many foods can actually prevent the formation of kidney stones, and pathologies of the kidneys. Fruits and vegetables and other foods rich in antioxidants can also prevent the onset of kidney cancer and help maintain healthy blood pressure. <u>Cranberries and lemons</u> protect kidney function by blocking the formation of <u>kidney stones</u> and also help to prevent urinary tract infections (UTIs). Many studies now confirm that consumption of cranberry juices and cranberry extracts breaks down and prevents the formation of calcium-rich deposits that form kidney stones. Cranberries also contain compounds that prevent the adhesion of bacteria to the inner epithelial lining of the urinary tract. This may explain how cranberry protects against urinary tract infections.

LEG CRAMPS or RESTLESS LEG SYNDROME: Leg cramps at night are painful, sudden involuntary contraction of the muscles in your calf and the feet. Leg cramps typically occur as you begin to fall asleep or wake up and can last for up to 10 minutes.

Signs, Symptoms and Causes: The exact cause of leg cramps at night has not yet been determined. Common factors associated with nighttime leg cramps include dehydration, prolonged periods of sitting, overuse of the leg muscles, spending long periods standing on concrete floors. Medical conditions, such as diabetes, peripheral vascular disease, blood clots and endocrine disorders, can also cause leg cramps.

Nutritional Factors: Eating a diet that contains plenty of potassium, magnesium and calcium and vitamin A and E may help prevent nighttime leg cramps from developing. Foods high in **vitamin A** include: Cantaloupe, Apricots, Carrots and Carrot Juice, Sweet Potatoes, Butternut Squash, Dark Leafy Greens such as Kale. These greens are great in a salad or steamed as a side: and as a bonus they are also high in calcium. Kale provides the most vitamin A.

The kind of lettuce also matters when it comes to vitamin A content. Dark colorful lettuces provide the most vitamin A. Meats: Liver (Turkey liver) provides the most vitamin A and a teaspoon of Cod liver oil will provide 500IU), Dried Herbs: Parsley provides the most vitamin A followed by Basil, Marjoram.   Spices (e.g., Paprika, Red Pepper, Cayenne, Chili Powder.

Foods high in **potassium** are: bananas oranges, tomatoes sweet potatoes, beet greens, halibut and soybeans. **Magnesium** is an essential mineral required by the body for maintaining normal muscle and nerve function, keeping a healthy immune system, maintaining heart rhythm, and building strong bones and muscles. A deficiency in magnesium can lead to muscle spasms, diabetes, cardiovascular disease, high blood pressure, anxiety disorders, osteoporosis, and migraines. Conversely, consuming too much magnesium typically causes diarrhea as the body attempts to excrete the excess. The current DV for magnesium is 400mg.

 Foods high in magnesium are: Bran (Rice, Wheat, and Oat), Dried Herbs, Squash, Pumpkin, and Watermelon Seeds (Dried or Roasted), Cocoa Powder (Dark Chocolate), Flaxseed, Sesame Seeds, Brazil Nuts, Sunflower Seeds, Almonds and Cashews, Pine Nuts,

Molasses, Soybeans (Edamame), and Spinach. **Calcium** rich foods are dairy products, dark green vegetables, sardines, and salmon. **Vitamin E** rich foods are sunflower seeds, sunflower oil, almonds and turnip greens.

Alternative measures to relieve Leg Cramps. Several activities will help you relieve a nighttime leg cramp. Flex your foot up toward your head to stretch the muscle. Increase the circulation to your leg muscles with massage, a hot shower, a warm bath. Ice, when used in combination with massage, may also help relieve some of the pain.

Regular exercise and supportive shoes may also help decrease your leg cramps. Other ways to prevent leg cramps include drinking plenty of water, sleeping on your side and not tucking in your covers. Some leg cramps result from serious medical conditions.

MACULAR DEGENERATION, AGE RELATED: Age-related macular degeneration (AMD) is a medical condition which usually affects older adults and results in a loss of vision in the center of the visual field (the macula) because of damage to the retina. It occurs in "dry" and "wet" forms. Macular Degeneration is a major cause of blindness and visual impairment in older adults (>50 years). Macular degeneration can make it difficult or impossible to read or recognize faces, although enough peripheral vision remains to allow other activities of daily life.

Starting from the inside of the eye and going towards the back, the three main layers at the back of the eye are the retina, which contains the nerves: the choroid, which contains the blood supply: and the sclera, which is the white of the eye. The macula is the central area of the retina, which provides the most detailed central vision. In the dry (nonexudative) form, cellular debris called drusen accumulates between the retina and the choroid, and the retina can become detached.

In the wet (exudative) form, which is more severe, blood vessels grow up from the choroid behind the retina, and the retina can also become detached. It can be treated with laser coagulation, and with medication that stops and sometimes reverses the growth of blood vessels.

Age-related macular degeneration begins with characteristic yellow deposits (drusen) in the macula, between the retinal pigment epithelium and the underlying choroid. The risk is higher when the drusen are large and numerous and associated with disturbance in the pigmented cell layer under the macula.

Large and soft drusen are related to elevated cholesterol deposits and may respond to cholesterol-lowering agents pharmacological agents as well as oranges, grapefruit and/or niacin). Dry AMD results from atrophy of the retinal pigment epithelial layer below the retina, which causes vision loss through loss of photoreceptors (rods and cones) in the central part of the eye.

No medical or surgical treatment is available for this condition, however vitamin supplements with high doses of antioxidants, (lutein and zeaxanthin) and/or foods containing high doses of lutein and zeaxanthin, have been suggested by the National Eye Institute to slow the progression of dry macular degeneration and, in some patients, and improve visual acuity. Macular degeneration is not painful, which may allow it to go unnoticed for some time.

Signs and symptoms of macular degeneration include: Normal vision at first then Blurred vision, Loss of color vision, Drusens, Pigmentary alterations, and Exudative changes (hemorrhages) in the eye. Visual acuity may drastically decrease (two levels or more), e.g.: 20/20 to 20/80.

Causes: <u>Aging</u>: Approximately 10% of patients 66 to 74 years of age will have findings of macular degeneration. *Drusen are similar in molecular composition to plaques and deposits in other age-related diseases such as Alzheimer's disease and atherosclerosis.* <u>Hypertension and Elevated Cholesterol</u> may increase the risk of AMD. <u>Abdominal obesity</u> is a risk factor, especially among men. Consuming high amounts of certain fats likely contributes to AMD, while monounsaturated fats are potentially protective.

In particular, <u>Omega-3 fatty acids may decrease the risk of AMD</u>. <u>Oxidative stress</u> is a major cause of age-related accumulation of low-molecular-weight, phototoxic, pro-oxidant melanin oligomers within lysosomes in the retinal pigment epithelium. <u>Race</u>: Macular degeneration is more likely to be found in Caucasians than in people of African descent. <u>Exposure to sunlight</u>. Evidence is conflicting as to whether exposure to sunlight contributes to the development of macular degeneration.

<u>Other research</u>, however, has shown high-energy visible light may contribute to AMD. <u>Smoking tobacco</u> increases the risk of AMD by two to three times that of someone who has never smoked, and may be the most important modifiable factor in its prevention. The role of retinal oxidative stress in the etiology of AMD by causing further inflammation of the macula is suggested by the enhanced rate of disease in smokers and those exposed to UV irradiation.

Nutritional factors: Some evidence supports a reduction in the risk of AMD with increasing intake of anti-oxidants: carotenoids, lutein and zeaxanthin, as well as consuming omega-3 fatty acids (DHA & EPA) and low glycemic index foods (low sugar content) has been correlated with a reduced progression of AMD. Avoid artificial non-nutritive sweeteners and trans-fats. Trans-fats are technically hydrogenated oils. The two popular hydrogenated oils are margarine and shortening.

MENOPAUSE: The word "menopause" literally means the "end of monthly cycles" from the Greek word pausis (cessation) and the root "men"- (month). The word "menopause" was created to describe this change in human females, where the end of fertility is traditionally indicated by the permanent stopping of monthly menses or menstruation. Menopause is the permanent cessation of the functions of the ovaries: i.e., the ripening and release of ova and the release of hormones that cause both the creation of the uterine lining and the subsequent shedding of the uterine lining (a.k.a. the menses or the "period").

Menopause itself, is a natural life change, not a disease state or a disorder. Menopause typically (but not always) occurs in women in midlife, during their late 40s or early 50s, and signals the end of the fertile phase of a woman's life. The transition from reproductive to non-reproductive is the result of a reduction in female hormonal production by the ovaries. Adult women who have their ovaries removed however, go immediately into surgical menopause, no matter how young they are.

Menopause is an unavoidable change that every woman will experience, assuming she reaches middle age and beyond. Menopause has a wide starting range, but can usually be expected in the age range of 42–58. An early menopause can be related to cigarette smoking, higher body mass index, racial and ethnic factors, illnesses, chemotherapy, radiation and the surgical removal of the ovaries, with or without the removal of the uterus. Menopause can be officially declared (in an adult woman who is not pregnant, is not lactating, and who has an intact uterus) when there has been amenorrhea (absence of any menstruation) for one complete year.

Signs and symptoms: There are many signs that lead up to menopause and many of which may extend well beyond it too. These include: vascular instability, hot flashes or hot flushes, night sweats and, in a few people, cold flashes, increased risk of Atherosclerosis, migraine, rapid heartbeat, urogenital atrophy (vaginal atrophy), atrophic vaginitis (thinning of the membranes of the vulva, the vagina, the cervix, and also the outer urinary tract), along with considerable shrinking and loss in elasticity of all of the outer and inner genital areas, itching, dryness, irregular bleeding at times, Watery discharge, urinary frequency, urinary incontinence, urinary urgency, increased susceptibility to inflammation and infection, e.g., vaginal candidiasis, and urinary tract infections.

Also, back pain, joint pain, muscle pain, osteopenia and the risk of osteoporosis gradually developing over time, breast atrophy, breast tenderness +/- swelling, decreased elasticity of the skin, <u>formication</u> (itching, tingling, burning, pins and needles, or sensation of ants crawling on or under the skin), skin thinning and becoming drier, psychological disturbance, i.e., depression and/or anxiety, fatigue, irritability, memory loss, and problems with concentration, mood disturbance, sleep disturbances, poor quality sleep, light sleep, insomnia and sleepiness, sexual disturbances, i.e., dyspareunia (Painful Intercourse), decreased libido, problems reaching orgasm, vaginal dryness and vaginal atrophy.

The only sign or effect that all women universally have in common is that by the end of the menopause transition every woman will have a complete cessation of menses. Women who have undergone hysterectomy with ovary conservation go through menopause on average 3.7 years earlier than the expected age. Menopause is perhaps most easily understood as the opposite process to menarche, the start of the monthly periods. However, menopause in women cannot satisfactorily be defined simply as the permanent "stopping of the monthly periods", because in reality what is happening to the uterus is quite secondary to the process: <u>it is what is happening to the ovaries</u> that is the crucial factor.

As an illustration of the central role that the ovaries play, it is worth pointing out that when for medical reasons the uterus has to be surgically removed (hysterectomy) in a younger woman, her periods will of course cease permanently, and the woman will be incapable of pregnancy, but as long as at least one of her ovaries is still functioning, the woman will not have reached true menopause.

Even without the presence of the uterus, ovulation and the release of the sequence of reproductive hormones will continue to cycle on, until "true" menopause is reached. In contrast to this, in circumstances where a woman's ovaries are removed (oophorectomy), even if the uterus were to be left intact, the woman will immediately be in "surgical menopause".

Surgical menopause is a menopause which is induced both suddenly and totally, by removal of both ovaries prior to the age of natural menopause. The term post-menopause is applied to women who have not experienced a menstrual bleed for a minimum of 12 months, assuming that they do still have a uterus, and are not pregnant or lactating. In women without a uterus, menopause or post-menopause is identified by a very high FSH level. At the point when a woman of menopausal age has had no periods or spotting for 12 months, she is considered to be one year into post-menopause.

Causes: Natural or physiological menopause occurs as a part of a woman's normal aging process. It is the result of the eventual depletion of almost all of the oocytes and ovarian follicles in the ovaries. This causes an increase in circulating follicle stimulating hormone (FSH) and luteinizing hormone (LH) levels because there are a decreased number of oocytes and follicles responding to these hormones and therefore a decrease in estrogen. This decrease in the production of estrogen leads to the peri-menopausal symptoms of hot flashes, insomnia and mood changes.

Nutritional info: It is important to examine the claim that herbal remedies help relieve menopausal symptoms. Botanical sources, referred to as phyto-estrogens, do not simply mimic the effects of human steroidal estrogen but exhibit both similar and divergent actions. The ultimate actions of these phytonutrients in specific cells is determined by many factors including the relative levels of the estrogen receptors. Thus they have been described to act somewhat like selective estrogen receptor modulators. Effects vary according to the phytoestrogen studied, cell line, tissue, species and response being evaluated. There are regular claims that soy isoflavones are beneficial concerning some symptoms of menopause. Isoflavones are naturally occurring nutrients, and daidzein and genistein are the main isoflavones found in soy. Several studies indicate that only 25 to 30 percent of the adult population of Western countries produces S-equol after eating soy foods containing isoflavones. "Recent human clinical studies showed that S-equol provided as a standardized soygerm-based dietary supplement helped reduce menopausal symptoms, bone loss and crow's feet skin wrinkles in menopausal women. Other remedies include red clover isoflavone extracts and black cohosh.

Black cohosh (Cimicifuga racemosa, also known as Actaea racemosa) is a North American native plant. It has common usage internationally for the treatment of hot flushes and sweats experienced by postmenopausal women. Many women arrive at their menopause transition years without knowing anything about what they might expect, or when or how the process might happen, and how long it might take. Very often a woman has not been informed in any way about this stage of life: at least in the US, it may often be the case that she has received no information from her physician, or from her older female family members, or from her social group. In the US, there appears to be a lingering taboo which hangs over this subject.

Other therapies: Low-dose prescription vaginal estrogen products such as estrogen creams are generally a safe way to use estrogen topically, to help vaginal thinning and dryness problems while only minimally increasing the levels of estrogen in the bloodstream. In terms of managing hot flashes, lifestyle measures, such as drinking cold liquids, staying in cool rooms, using fans, removing excess clothing layers when a hot flash strikes.

MULTIPLE SCLEROSIS: Multiple sclerosis (MS), also known as "disseminated sclerosis" is <u>an inflammatory disease in which the fatty myelin sheaths around the axons of the brain and spinal cord are damaged</u>, leading to demyelination and scarring as well as a broad spectrum of signs and symptoms. Disease onset usually occurs in young adults, and it is more common in women. It has a prevalence that ranges between 2 and 150 per 100,000. **MS affects the ability of nerve cells in the brain and spinal cord to communicate with each other effectively**.

Nerve cells communicate by sending electrical signals called action potentials down long fibers called axons, which are contained within an insulating substance called myelin. <u>In MS, the body's own immune system attacks and damages the myelin</u>. When myelin is lost, the axons can no longer effectively conduct signals. The name multiple sclerosis refers to scars (scleroses-better known as plaques or lesions) particularly in the white matter of the brain and spinal cord, which is mainly composed of myelin.

Although much is known about the mechanisms involved in the disease process, the cause remains unknown. Theories include genetics or infections. Different environmental risk factors have also been found. <u>Almost any neurological symptom can appear</u>

with the disease, and often progresses to physical and cognitive disability.

MS takes several forms, with new symptoms occurring either in discrete attacks (relapsing forms) or slowly accumulating over time (progressive forms). Between attacks, symptoms may go away completely, but permanent neurological problems often occur, especially as the disease advances. There is no known cure for multiple sclerosis. **Treatments attempt to return function after an attack, prevent new attacks, and prevent disability.** MS medications can have adverse effects or be poorly tolerated, and many people pursue alternative treatments, despite the lack of supporting scientific study. The prognosis is difficult to predict: it depends mainly on the subtype of the disease, the individual's disease characteristics, the initial symptoms and the degree of disability the person experiences as time advances. Life expectancy of people with MS is 5 to 10 years shorter than that of the unaffected population.

Signs and Symptoms: A person with MS can suffer almost any neurological symptom or sign, including changes in sensation such as loss of sensitivity or tingling, pricking or numbness (hypoesthesia and paresthesia), muscle weakness, clonus, muscle spasms, or difficulty in moving: difficulties with coordination and balance (ataxia): problems in speech (dysarthria) or swallowing (dysphagia), visual problems (nystagmus, optic neuritis including phosphenes, or diplopia), fatigue, acute or chronic pain, and bladder and bowel difficulties.

Cognitive impairment of varying degrees and emotional symptoms of depression or unstable mood are also common. Uhthoff's phenomenon, an exacerbation of extant symptoms due to an exposure to higher than usual ambient temperatures, and Lhermitte's sign, an electrical sensation that runs down the back when bending the neck, are particularly characteristic of MS although not specific. The main clinical measure of disability progression and symptom severity is the Expanded Disability Status Scale or EDSS. Symptoms of MS usually appear in episodic acute periods of worsening (called relapses, exacerbations, bouts, attacks, or "flare-ups"), in a gradually progressive deterioration of neurologic function, or in a combination of both.

Causes: Most likely MS occurs as a result of some combination of environmental conditions (pesticides, weather extremes), nutritional deficiencies (healthy fats and vitamin B & D and mineral deficiencies), genetic and infectious factors, and possibly other factors like vascular problems. Theories try to combine the known data into plausible explanations, but none has proved definitive.

Genetic Factors: People with changes in the HLA region of Chromosome 6 have increased probability of suffering MS. MS is not considered a hereditary disease. However, a number of genetic variations have been shown to increase the risk of developing the disease. The risk of acquiring MS is higher in relatives of a person with the disease than in the general population, especially in the case of siblings, parents, and children. The disease has an overall familial recurrence rate of 20%. In the case of monozygotic twins, concordance occurs only in about 35% of cases, while it goes down to around 5% in the case of siblings and even lower in half-siblings.

Environmental factors: Different environmental factors, both of infectious and non infectious origin have been proposed as risk factors for MS. MS is more common in people who live farther from the equator, although many exceptions exist. Decreased sunlight exposure has been linked with a higher risk of MS. Decreased vitamin D production and intake has been the main biological mechanism used to explain the higher risk among those less exposed to sun. Severe stress may be a risk factor although evidence is weak. Smoking has also been shown to be an independent risk factor for developing MS. Association with occupational exposures and toxins—mainly solvents—has been evaluated, but no clear conclusions have been reached. Vaccinations were investigated as causal factors for the disease: but, most studies show no association between MS and vaccines. Several other possible risk factors, such as diet and hormone intake, have been investigated: however, evidence on their relation with the disease is "sparse and unpersuasive".

Infections: Many microbes have been proposed as potential infectious triggers of MS, but none have been substantiated. Evidence for viruses as a cause includes the presence of oligoclonal bands in the brain and cerebrospinal fluid of most people with MS, the association of several viruses with human demyelination encephalomyelitis, and induction of demyelination in animals through viral infection. Other diseases that have also been related with MS are measles, mumps, and rubella.

Multiple sclerosis and relapses are often unpredictable, occurring without warning and without obvious inciting factors with a rate rarely above one and a half per year. Some attacks, however, are preceded by common triggers. The disease as well as relapses occur more frequently during spring and summer. Viral infections such as the common cold, influenza, or gastroenteritis increase the risk of relapse. Stress may also trigger an attack. Pregnancy affects the susceptibility to relapse, with a lower relapse rate at each trimester of gestation. During the first few months after delivery, however, the risk of relapse is increased. Overall, pregnancy does not seem to influence long-term disability.

Treatment of multiple sclerosis: Although there is no known cure for multiple sclerosis, several therapies have proven helpful. The primary aims of therapy are returning function after an attack, preventing new attacks, and preventing disability. As with any medical treatment, medications used in the management of MS have several adverse effects. During symptomatic attacks, administration of high doses of intravenous <u>corticosteroids</u>, such as methyl-prednisolone, is the routine therapy for acute relapses. Although generally effective in the short term for relieving symptoms, corticosteroid treatments do not appear to have a significant impact on long-term recovery. Oral and intravenous administration seems to have similar efficacy. Consequences of severe attacks which do not respond to corticosteroids might be treated by <u>plasmapheresis</u>. Treatment with <u>interferons</u> during an initial attack can decrease the chance that a person will develop clinical MS.

<u>Management of the effects of MS</u>. Disease-modifying treatments reduce the progression rate of the disease, but do not stop it. Both drug therapy and neuro-rehabilitation have shown to ease the burden of some symptoms, though neither influences disease progression. Some symptoms have a good response to medication, such as unstable bladder and spasticity, while management of many others is much more complicated. As for any person with neurologic deficits, a multidisciplinary approach is key to improving quality of life: because individuals with MS may need help from almost any health profession or service at some point. Research has supported the rehabilitative role of physical activity in improving muscle power, mobility, mood, bowel health, general conditioning and quality of life. Care should be taken not to overheat a person with MS during the course of exercise. Activities may include resistance training, walking, swimming, yoga, tai chi, and others.

Nutritional factors: The right diet for someone with multiple sclerosis is simple--eat a varied diet filled with fruits, vegetables, lean proteins, unsaturated healthy fats such as omega 3 EPA and DHA, fiber and 8 to 10 glasses of water every day. There is no magic trick to what nutrition can do for you. The key is to take care of your body and give it all of the essential vitamins and minerals that it needs, limiting or avoid those foods that we all know aren't good for anyone (e.g., artificial non-nutritive sweeteners and trans-fats such a margarine and/or shortening and processed food products made with these man-made chemicals and hydrogenated oils. All healthy diets should incorporate omega 3 fatty acids since we are dealing with the myelin that covers nerves, foods that are high in omega 3 fatty acids: and again <u>avoid</u> all artificial non-nutritive sweeteners and bad fats, i.e. trans-fats, which are hydrogenated oils.

Alternative treatments: Alternative treatments are pursued by some people, despite the shortage of supporting, comparable, replicated scientific study. Examples are herbal medicine (including the use of medical cannabis) and hyperbaric oxygenation.

NON-ULCER DYSPEPSIA: Functional Dyspepsia or just Dyspepsia also known as upset stomach, indigestion, or heartburn -refers to a condition of impaired digestion. It is a medical condition characterized by chronic or recurrent pain in the upper abdomen, upper abdominal fullness and feeling full earlier than expected when eating. It can be accompanied by bloating, belching, nausea, or heartburn.

Dyspepsia is a common problem, and is frequently associated with, gastro-esophageal reflux disease (GERD) or gastritis. In a small minority it may be the first symptom of peptic ulcer disease (an ulcer of the stomach or duodenum) and occasionally cancer. Hence, unexplained new onset of dyspepsia in people over 55 or the presence of other alarming symptoms may require further investigations. Functional dyspepsia (previously called non-ulcer dyspepsia) is dyspepsia that is "without evidence of an organic disease that is likely to explain the symptoms". Functional dyspepsia is estimated to affect about 15% of the general population in western countries.

Signs and symptoms: The characteristic symptoms of dyspepsia are upper abdominal pain, bloating, fullness and tenderness on palpation. Important to note is the fact: "Pain worsened by exertion and associated with nausea and perspiration may also indicate angina i.e.," heart pain".

Occasionally dyspeptic symptoms are caused by medication: such as (1) calcium antagonists (used for angina or high blood pressure, i.e. cardiazem, nitrates (used for angina), (2) theophylline (used for chronic lung disease), (3) bisphosphonates, (used for osteoporosis), (4) "mycins" antibiotics (like erythromycin) used for infection, (5) non-steroidal anti-inflammatory drugs (i.e. NSAIDs) used for pain and (6) corticosteroids (dexamethasone, cortisone, prednisone) also used as pain as well as swelling and asthma and allergy relief.

 The presence of gastrointestinal bleeding, difficulty swallowing, loss of appetite, unintentional weight loss, abdominal swelling and persistent vomiting are suggestive of peptic ulcer disease or malignancy, and would necessitate urgent investigations.

Diagnosis: People over 55 years with recent onset dyspepsia or those with alarm symptoms should be urgently investigated by upper gastrointestinal endoscopy. This will rule out peptic ulcer disease, medication-related ulceration, malignancy and other rarer causes. People under the age of 55 years with no alarm features do not need endoscopy but are considered for investigation for peptic ulcer disease caused by Helicobacter pylori (H. pylori) infection.

 Investigation for H. pylori infection is usually performed when there is a moderate to high prevalence of this infection in the local community or the person with dyspepsia has other risk factors for H. pylori infection, i.e., immigration from a high prevalence area or ethnicity. If infection is confirmed it can usually be eradicated by medication. Medication-related dyspepsia is usually related to non-steroidal anti-inflammatory drugs (NSAIDs) and bisphosphonates

(Fosamax). These medicines can cause bleeding or ulceration with perforation of stomach wall.

Treatment: Functional and undifferentiated dyspepsia have similar treatments. Decisions around the use of drug therapy are difficult because trials included heartburn in the definition of dyspepsia. This led to the results favoring (PPIs) <u>proton pump inhibitors i.e., *Prilosec (Omeprazole), Prevacid (Lanzoprazole)*, etc., which are more effective for the treatment of heartburn</u>.

Traditional therapies used for this diagnosis include lifestyle modification, antacids: i.e., *Maalox, Mylanta, Tums,* etc., H2-receptor antagonists: i.e., *Tagamet (Cimetidine), Zantac (Ranitidine), Pepcid (Famotidine)*, etc., prokinetic agents: i.e., *Metaclopromide (Reglan)* and antiflatulents: i.e., *Simethicone (Mylicon)*.

It has been noted that one of the most frustrating aspects of treating functional dyspepsia is that these traditional agents have been shown to have little or no efficacy. Antacids and *Sucralfate* were found to be no better than placebo in a literature review. Modern prokinetic agents such as *Metoclopramide (Reglan)*, and *Cisapride (Propulsid)* have little or no established efficacy and often result in substantial side effects. Simethicone has been found to be of some value. A 2002 systemic review of herbal products found that several herbs, including <u>peppermint</u> and <u>caraway seed</u> (also known as meridian fennel, or Persian cumin), have anti-dyspeptic effects for non-ulcer dyspepsia with "encouraging safety profiles".

The herbal extract, **_Iberogast_**, (also known as STW5, is a liquid formulation of nine herbs. Named after the genus (Iberis) of one of its ingredients, it is also claimed to possess anti-inflammatory, antioxidative and free radical-inhibiting properties as well as <u>reduce gastric acid secretion</u>) was significantly more effective than placebo at treating patients with functional dyspepsia through the targeting of multiple dyspeptic pathologies. This German-made phytopharmaceutical (1961) was found to be equivalent to *Cisapride (Propulsid)* and significantly superior to *Metoclopramide (Reglan)* at reducing the symptoms of functional dyspepsia over a four week period.

Nutritional Factors: <u>Red pepper powder</u> along with <u>ginger</u> and related products made from them have been shown to have some positive results in alleviating symptom of dyspepsia: in particular for motion sickness and nausea. Also, foods that contain <u>flavonoids, such as apples, celery, cranberries, and cranberry juice</u> may inhibit the growth of Helicobacter pylori, the bacteria that is responsible for most stomach ulcers. Chewing food thoroughly can help control symptoms of dyspepsia. Eating in a leisurely, calm and relaxed atmosphere and chewing and swallowing foods slowly may help reduce symptoms of dyspepsia. Taking steps to reduce excess gas and belching may also help control symptoms of dyspepsia. To avoid taking in excessive air, avoid smoking, eating quickly, chewing gum, drinking through a straw and drinking carbonated beverages.

<u>Ulcers are not caused by spicy food or stress, but are caused by H. pylori or long-term use of nonsteroidal anti-inflammatory drugs.</u>

However, some foods may trigger dyspepsia. These foods may include fatty, fried, carbonated beverages, caffeinated and decaffeinated coffee and tea, alcohol, cocoa, chocolate, citrus fruits and juices, and tomato products. These foods can increase stomach acid. Keep track of foods that cause symptoms or dyspepsia and omit any food that causes discomfort. If a peptic ulcer is suspected, medication is almost always needed to heal or alleviate symptoms and must be used to treat the H. pylori. An empty stomach can sometimes produce dyspepsia symptoms. Consuming six small meals a day as opposed to three larger meals may help with symptoms, as can avoiding skipping meals. Eating within two hours before bedtime may also trigger symptoms of acid reflux or dyspepsia.

OBESITY: Obesity is a leading preventable cause of death worldwide. With increasing prevalence of obesity in adults and children, authorities view obesity as one of the most serious public health problems of the 21st century. Obesity has become a medical problem. Also, obesity is a disease process, in which excess body fat has accumulated to the extent that it may have an adverse effect on health, leading to decreased quality of life, reduced life expectancy and/or increased health problems.

It is defined by body mass index (BMI) and further evaluated in terms of fat distribution via the waist–hip ratio and cardiovascular risk factors. BMI is closely related to both percentage body fat and total body fat. People are considered as obese when their body mass index (BMI), exceeds 30 kg/m2. BMI is calculated by dividing the subject's mass by the square of his or her height, typically expressed in metric units: (Metric: BM I= kilograms /meters squared). The World Health Organization (WHO), provided the values listed in the table below.

BMI	Classification
• < 18.5	underweight
• 18.5–24.9	normal weight
• 25.0–29.9	overweight
• 30.0–34.9	class I obesity
• 35.0–39.9	class II obesity

The surgical literature breaks down "class III" obesity into further   categories whose exact values are still disputed.
- Any BMI ≥ 35 or 40 is severe obesity
- A BMI of ≥ 35 or 40–45 is morbid obesity
- A BMI of ≥ 45 or 50 is super morbid obesity

Effects on health: Excessive body weight is associated with various diseases and in many cases actually causes medical disease, particularly cardiovascular diseases, diabetes mellitus type 2, obstructive sleep apnea, certain types of cancer, and osteoarthritis to mention a few. Obesity has been found to reduce life expectancy.

A BMI above 32 has been associated with a doubled mortality rate among women over a 16-year period. In the United States, obesity is estimated to cause an excess 100,000 to 365,000 deaths per year. On average, obesity reduces life expectancy by four to ten years: a BMI of 30–35 reduces life expectancy by two to four years, while severe obesity (BMI > 40) reduces life expectancy by 10 years.

Morbidity or incidences of ill health: Obesity increases the risk of many physical and mental conditions. The most common medical disorder associated with obesity is **insulin resistance or the metabolic syndrome. This syndrome includes heart disease and diabetes as well as many more age related metabolic medical diseases.** The Metabolic Syndrome, is also known as Insulin Resistance Syndrome. It is a combination of medical disorders that are related to the body's inability to metabolize insulin correctly.

Some of these medical disorders include: obesity, type 2 diabetes mellitus, high blood pressure, high blood cholesterol, and high triglyceride levels, heart disease, kidney disease, eye diseases, neurological diseases, sleep apnea, and some cancers, etc. Many of the complications are either directly caused by obesity or indirectly related through mechanisms sharing a common cause such as a poor diet or a sedentary lifestyle or damaged insulin receptors. The strength of the link between obesity and specific conditions varies. One of the strongest is the link with type 2 diabetes.

Excess body fat underlies 64% of cases of diabetes in men and 77% of cases in women. Health consequences fall into two broad categories: (1) those attributable to the effects of increased fat mass (size and weight of fat): such as osteoarthritis, obstructive sleep apnea, social stigmatization and (2) those due to the increased number of fat cells (diabetes, cancer, cardiovascular disease, non-alcoholic fatty liver disease). Increases in body fat alter the body's response to insulin, potentially leading to insulin resistance or the metabolic syndrome. Increased fat also creates a prothrombotic (blood clot) state and a proinflammatory state (arthritis. It is this proinflammatory state that leads to most of the metabolic diseases listed below.

Medical conditions affected by an over-weight are as follows by medical specialty.

Cardiology: Ischemic heart disease: angina and myocardial infarction, Congestive heart failure, High blood pressure, Abnormal cholesterol levels, Deep vein thrombosis and pulmonary embolism
Dermatology: Stretch marks, Acanthosis nigricans, Lymphedema, Cellulitis, Hirsutism, Intertrigo
Endocrinology and Reproductive medicine: Diabetes mellitus, Polycystic ovarian syndrome, Menstrual disorders, Infertility, Complications during pregnancy, Birth defects, Intrauterine fetal death
Gastrointestinal: Gastroesophageal reflux disease, Fatty liver disease, Cholelithiasis (gallstones).
Neurology: Stroke, Migraines, Carpal tunnel syndrome, Dementia/Alzheimer's disease, Multiple sclerosis
Oncology (Cancer): Breast, ovarian, Esophageal, colorectal, Liver, pancreatic, Gallbladder, stomach. Endometrial, cervical, Prostate, kidney, Non-Hodgkin's lymphoma, multiple myeloma.
Psychiatry: Depression, Social stigmatization
Respirology: Obstructive sleep apnea, Obesity hypoventilation syndrome, Asthma, Increased complications during general anaesthesia.
Rheumatology and Orthopedics: Gout, Poor mobility, Osteoarthritis, Low back pain.

Urology and Nephrology: Erectile dysfunction, Urinary incontinence, Chronic renal failure, Hypogonadism, Buried penis syndrome

Causes of Obesity at an <u>individual level</u> are the result of a combination of excessive food calorie intake and a lack of physical activity. A limited number of cases are due primarily to genetics, medical reasons, or psychiatric illness.

Causes of obesity at a <u>societal level</u> are felt to be due to an easily accessible and palatable high glycemic (especially sweet tasting food) diets, increased reliance on cars, and mechanized manufacturing. A 2006 review identified nine other possible contributors to the recent increase of obesity: (1) endocrine disruptors (environmental pollutants that interfere with lipid metabolism), (2) insufficient sleep, (3) decreased variability in ambient temperature, (4) decreased rates of smoking, because smoking suppresses appetite, (5) increased use of medications that can cause weight gain (e.g., atypical antipsychotics), (6) proportional increases in ethnic and age groups that tend to be heavier, (7) epigenetic risk factors passed on generationally, (8) natural selection for higher BMI, and (9) assortative mating leading to increased concentration of obesity risk factors (this would increase the number of obese people by increasing population variance in weight).

Treatment. <u>Dieting and physical exercise are the mainstays of treatment for obesity</u>. (1) Diet quality can be improved by reducing the consumption of energy-dense foods such as those high in fat and sugars, and by increasing the intake of dietary fiber of natural (unprocessed fruits and vegetables. Anti-obesity drugs may be taken to reduce appetite or inhibit fat absorption together with a suitable diet. If diet, exercise and medication are not effective, a gastric balloon may assist with weight loss, or surgery may be performed to reduce stomach volume and/or bowel length, leading to earlier satiation and reduced ability to absorb nutrients from food.

Diet: Total calorie consumption has been found to be related to obesity. The per capita dietary energy supply varies markedly between different regions and countries. It has also changed significantly over time. From the early 1970s to the late 1990s the average calories available per person per day (the amount of food bought) increased in all parts of the world except Eastern Europe. The United States had the highest availability with 2,854 calories per person in 1996. This increased further in 2003 to 3,754.

Most of this extra food calories came from an increase in carbohydrate consumption rather than fat or protein consumption. The primary sources of these extra carbohydrates are sweetened beverages, which now account for greatest source of daily food energy in young adults in America: potato chip snacks are second. Consumption of sweetened drinks (especially those sweetened with high fructose corn syrup) is believed to be the main source of calories contributing to the rising rates of obesity.

In the United States sugar prices are two to three times higher than in the rest of the world, which makes HFCS significantly cheaper, so that it is the principal sweetener used in processed foods and beverages. It is commonly used in breads, cereals, breakfast bars, lunch meats, yogurts, soups, and condiments. The widespread availability of nutritional guidelines has done little to address the problems of overeating and poor dietary choice.

(2) Sedentary lifestyle: A sedentary lifestyle plays a significant role in obesity. Worldwide there has been a large shift towards less physically demanding work, and currently at least 60% of the world's population gets insufficient exercise. This is primarily due to increasing use of mechanized transportation and a greater prevalence of labor-saving technology in the home. In children,

there appear to be declines in levels of physical activity due to less walking and physical education. In both children and adults, there is an association between computer work or pastime and television viewing time and the risk of obesity. A review found 63 of 73 studies (86%) showed an increased rate of childhood obesity with increased media exposure, with rates increasing proportionally to time spent watching television or on line socializing.

(3) Genetics of obesity: Like many other medical conditions, obesity is the result of an interplay between genetic and environmental factors. Polymorphisms in various genes controlling appetite and metabolism predispose to obesity but only when sufficient food calories are present. As of 2006 more than 41 of these sites have been linked to the development of obesity when a favorable environment is present. People with two copies of the FMO gene (fat mass and obesity gene) has been found on average to weigh 6 to 10 more and have a 1.67-fold greater risk of obesity compared to those without the risk allele (gene). The percentage of obesity that can be attributed to genetics varies, depending on the population examined.

 Obesity is a major feature in several syndromes, such as Prader-Willi syndrome, Bardet-Biedl syndrome, and Cohen syndrome. Studies that have focused upon inheritance patterns rather than upon specific genes have found that 80% of the offspring of two obese parents were obese, in contrast to less than 10% of the offspring of two parents who were of normal weight.

Other illnesses: Certain physical and mental illnesses and the pharmaceutical substances used to treat them can increase risk of obesity. **Certain medications** may cause weight gain or changes in body composition: these include insulin, sulfonylureas, thiazolidinediones, atypical antipsychotics, antidepressants, steroids, certain anticonvulsants e.g., phenytoin and valproate, and some forms of hormonal contraception. Medical illnesses that increase obesity risk include several rare genetic syndromes (listed above) as well as some congenital or acquired conditions such as: Cushing's syndrome, Hypothyroidism, Growth hormone deficiency. Also eating disorders such as: binge eating disorder and night eating syndrome.

Obesity is not regarded as a psychiatric disorder. However, the risk of overweight and obesity is higher in patients with psychiatric disorders than in persons without psychiatric disorders.

 Social determinants of obesity: While genetic influences are important to understanding obesity, they cannot explain the current dramatic increase seen within specific countries or globally. Though it is accepted that calorie consumption in excess of energy expenditure leads to obesity on an individual basis, the cause of the shifts in these two factors on the societal scale is much debated.

 There are a number of theories as to the cause but most believe it is a combination of various factors. The correlation between social class and BMI varies globally. A review in 1989 found that in developed countries women of a high social class were less likely to be obese. No significant differences were seen among men of different social classes. Many explanations have been put forth for associations between BMI and social class. It is thought that in developed countries, the wealthy are able to afford more nutritious food, they are under greater social pressure to remain slim, and have more opportunities along with greater expectations for physical fitness. In undeveloped countries the ability to afford food, high energy expenditure with physical labor, and cultural values favoring a larger body size are believed to contribute to the observed patterns.

Attitudes toward body mass held by people in one's life may also play a role in obesity. A correlation in BMI changes over time has been found among friends, siblings, and spouses. Stress and perceived low social status appear to increase the risk of obesity. Smoking has a significant effect on an individual's weight. Those who quit smoking gain an average of 4.4 kilograms (9.7 lb) for men and 5.0 kilograms (11.0 lb) for women over ten years.

 Malnutrition in early life is believed to play a role in the rising rates of obesity in the developing world. Endocrine changes that occur during periods of malnutrition may promote the storage of fat once more food calories becomes available. Consistent with cognitive epidemiological data, numerous studies confirm that obesity is associated with cognitive deficits. Whether obesity causes cognitive deficits, or vice versa is unclear at present.

 Pathophysiology: There are many possible pathophysiological mechanisms involved in the development and/or the maintenance of obesity. This field of research had been almost unapproached until leptin (a hormone) was discovered in 1994. Since this discovery, many other hormonal mechanisms have been elucidated that participate in the regulation of appetite and food intake, storage patterns of adipose tissue, and development of insulin resistance. Since leptin was discovery, ghrelin, insulin, orexin, PYY 3-36, cholecystokinin, adiponectin, as well as many other mediators have been studied. The adipokines are mediators produced by adipose tissue: their action is thought to modify many obesity-related diseases. Leptin and ghrelin are considered to be complementary in their influence on appetite, with ghrelin produced by the stomach modulating short-term appetitive control (i.e. to eat when the stomach is empty and to stop when the stomach is full or stretched). Leptin is produced by adipose tissue to signal fat storage reserves in the body, and mediates long-term appetitive controls (i.e. to eat more when fat storages are low and eat less when fat storages are high).

Although administration of leptin may be effective in a small subset of obese individuals who are leptin deficient (store fat more readily), most obese individuals are thought to be "leptin resistant" because they have been found to have high levels of leptin. This resistance is thought to explain in part why administration of leptin has not been shown to be effective in suppressing appetite in most obese people.

While leptin and ghrelin are produced peripherally, they control appetite through their actions on the central nervous system. In particular, they and other appetite-related hormones act on the hypothalamus, a region of the brain central to the regulation of food intake and energy expenditure.

Note: when ghrelin is high your become hungry and are likely to gain weight and when leptin in high you are more like to lose weight and of course the reverse is just as true. Public health: The World Health Organization (WHO) predicts that overweight and obesity may soon replace more traditional public health concerns such as under-nutrition and infectious diseases as the most significant cause of poor health.

Obesity is a public health problem and a public policy problem because everyone is affected by its prevalence, costs, and negative health effects. Public health efforts are now seeking to understand and correct the environmental factors responsible for the increasing prevalence of obesity in the population. Solutions look at changing the factors that cause excess food calorie consumption and inhibit physical activity. Efforts include federally reimbursed meal programs in schools, limiting direct junk food marketing to children, and decreasing access to sugar-sweetened beverages in schools. When constructing urban environments, efforts have been made to increase access to parks and to develop pedestrian routes.

Management of obesity: The main treatment for obesity remains and consists of dieting and physical exercise. Diet programs may produce weight loss over the short term, but maintaining this weight loss is frequently difficult and often requires making exercise and a lower food calorie diets a permanent part of a person's lifestyle. Success rates of long-term weight loss maintenance with lifestyle changes are low, ranging from 2–20%.

Weight loss however is modest with an average of 6.4 lb at 1 to 4 years and there is little information on how weight loss drugs affect longer-term complications of obesity. Two new weight loss medications are now available. Lorcaserin (Belviq) results in an average 6 lb weight loss (3% of body mass) greater than placebo over a year. A combination of phentermine and topiramate (Qsymia) is also somewhat effective. The most effective treatment for obesity is surgery. Surgery for severe obesity is associated with long-term weight loss and decreased overall mortality.

The Greeks were the first to recognize obesity as a medical disorder.

Hippocrates wrote that "Corpulence is not only a disease itself, but the harbinger of others." Note: Before the 20th century, obesity was rare: however, in 1997 the WHO formally recognized obesity as a global epidemic. <u>Childhood obesity</u>: Changing diet and decreasing physical activity are believed to be the two most important causes of childhood obesity. Because childhood obesity often persists into adulthood and is associated with numerous chronic illnesses, children who are obese are often tested for hypertension, diabetes, hyperlipidemia, and fatty liver. Treatments used in children are primarily lifestyle interventions and behavioral techniques. In the United States, medications are not FDA approved for use in this age group.

Nutritional factors: Reducing calories and eating healthier <u>are vital</u> to overcoming obesity. Although you may lose weight quickly at first, slow and steady weight loss of 1 or 2 pounds (1/2 to 1 kilogram) a week over the long term is considered the safest way to lose weight and the best way to keep it off permanently. Avoid drastic and unrealistic diet changes, such as crash diets, because they're unlikely to help you keep excess weight off for the long term. Dietary ways to overcome obesity include:

A low-calorie diet. The key to weight loss is reducing high glycemic food calories . Those are calories found in sweets and bread products. You can review your typical eating and drinking habits to see how many calories you normally consume and where you can cut back. You can decide how many calories you need to take in each day to lose weight, but a typical amount is 1,000 to 1,600 calories -total.

 Feeling full on less. The concept of "energy dense foods" can help you satisfy your hunger with fewer calories. All foods have a certain number of calories within a given amount (volume). Some foods, such as desserts, candies, fats and processed foods, are high in "energy density". This means that a small volume of that food has a large number of calories. In contrast, other foods, such as fruits and vegetables (most vegetable salads), have low "energy density". These foods provide a larger portion size with a fewer number of calories. By eating larger portions of foods less packed with calories, you reduce hunger pangs, take in fewer calories and feel full and better about your meal, which contributes to how satisfied you feel overall.

Adopting a healthy-eating plan. To make your overall diet healthier, eat more plant-based foods, such as fruits, vegetables and whole-grain carbohydrates (oatmeal). Also emphasize lean sources of protein, such as beans, lentils and soy, and lean meats. Try to include fish twice a week. Limit salt and added sugar. Stick with low-fat dairy products. Eat small amounts of fats, and make sure they come from heart-healthy sources, such as nuts and olive, canola and nut oils.

Meal replacements. These plans suggest that you replace one or two meals with "their" products — such as low-calorie shakes or meal bars — and eat healthy snacks and a healthy, balanced third meal that's low in fat and calories. In the short term, this type of diet can help you lose weight. Keep in mind that these diets likely won't teach you how to change your overall lifestyle, so you may have to keep this up if you want to keep your weight off.

 Be wary of quick fixes. You may be tempted by fad diets that promise fast and easy weight loss. The reality, however, is that there are no magic foods or quick fixes. Fad diets may help in the short term, but the long-term results don't appear to be any better than other diets. Similarly, you may lose weight on a crash diet, but you're likely to regain it when you stop the diet. To lose weight and keep it off you have to adopt healthy-eating habits that you can maintain over time. The Keto-Genic Diet is a modified "Atkins" diet. Weight loss is safe and just as effective on this diet.

KETO-GENIC DIET

Menu: <u>Breakfast</u>: 2eggs any style, bacon, cheese (add a vinegar tablet or ½ grapefruit   or ½ cup grapefruit juice). 1 to 2 cups Tea or Coffee [black - no sugar (no artificial sweeteners)].

 <u>Lunch or Dinner/Supper</u>: Meat: beef hamburgers or steak, chicken, fish, pork, (broiled, baked or grilled): Salad with vinegar & oil – may have fruit and nuts on salad: Vegetables-raw or cooked in real butter or canola oil. 2 to 3 cups or glasses of un-sweet Tea or Black Coffee.

1.	At meal time eat until you are full: this distends the stomach and stops the production of <u>Ghrelin</u>: a hormone that triggers the brain you are starving. <u>Ghrelin is the hunger hormone</u>.

2.	Do not eliminate the "real fat" portions from this diet. Real fat does not form fat directly because it does not raise insulin. (**Insulin is the fat storing hormone: Glucagon is the fat burning hormone.**)

3.	This diet completely eliminates simple carbohydrates and sugars: the real fat formers because they signal the pancreas to release a surge of - **insulin: the fat storing hormone**.

4.	Grapefruit or vinegar tablets or dill pickles are an important aspect of this diet: These foods act as catalysts that start the fat burning process - (Lipolysis).

5.	Do not eat deserts, breads, potatoes and white vegetables. These are considered high glycemic foods. They cause a surge in Insulin: which actually causes weight gain. You may double the helpings of meat or salad or other low-glycemic foods. Eat until you are full: but stay away from high glycemic foods.

6.   You may snack on raw unsalted nuts or raw vegetables, etc. However, if you eat the combination of foods suggested you will not get hungry.

7.   Drink 8 cups (8 oz) of unflavored water every day. (This is ½ gallon of pure water).

<u>Water neutralizes the sugar or sweet flavor on your tongue</u> and thus decreases the production of a surge of insulin. Water also helps eliminate body waste faster preventing constipation. Constipation can interfere with healthy weight loss.

You may have: Broccoli, Carrots, Cabbage, Cole slaw, Cucumbers, Radishes, Spinach, Tomatoes, Lettuce, Nuts (no salt), Squash, Fried green vegetables, Green beans, Beans, Green apples, Grapes, Berries (black, blue or strawberries), Pears, Plums, Mangos, Mustard, Peppers, Real Dressing, Garlic and herbal seasoning, Tuna, Sardines, Salmon, Bacon, Meats, Chili (no beans), Cheese, Skim milk, and Hot Oatmeal with butter but no sweetener. **NOTE:** Use Grapefruit or Grapefruit juice or Vinegar tablets or Dill pickles with each meal.

You may not have: Highly processed Cereal, Corn, Sweet Pickles, Jam or Jelly, Canned fruits in heavy syrup, Fruit Juices that contain artificial sweeteners and/or high fructose corn syrup, Diet Dressing, White Onions, Peas, Pasta, Pretzels, Potatoes, Potato Chips, Corn Chips, Sweet Pickles, and all sweet desserts while on the Keto-Genic Diet.

 <u>This diet works best if you are will go on a "sugar-salt fast" the first two weeks.</u> You can go off this recommended low glycemic diet – above- one day every other week and still lose weight.

OSTEOPOROSIS and OSTEOARTHRITIS: Osteoporosis ("porous bones") is a disease of bones that leads to an increased risk of fracture. In osteoporosis, the bone mineral density (BMD) is reduced, bone micro-architecture deteriorates, and the amount and variety of proteins in bone are altered. <u>Osteoporosis is defined by the World Health Organization (WHO) as a bone mineral density that is 2.5 standard deviations or more below the mean peak bone mass (average of young, healthy adults) as measured by DEXA.</u>

The disease may be classified as (primary) type 1, or (secondary) type 2. The form of osteoporosis most common in women after menopause is referred to as primary type 1 or postmenopausal osteoporosis. When there is no known cause this disease process is referred to as primary type 1 osteoarthritis. When the cause of the osteoarthritis is known, the condition is referred to as secondary type 2 osteoarthritis. Osteoarthritis is a form of arthritis that features the breakdown and eventual loss of the cartilage of one or more joints.

Osteoarthritis is joint inflammation that results from loss of cartilage due to cartilage degeneration. Cartilage is a protein substance that serves as a "cushion" between the bones of the joints. Osteoarthritis is abbreviated as OA or referred to as degenerative arthritis or degenerative joint disease (DJD). Osteoarthritis commonly affects the hands, feet, spine, and large weight-bearing joints, such as (i.e.) the hips and knees. The goal of treatment in osteoarthritis is to reduce joint pain and inflammation while improving and maintaining joint function.

Causes: Osteoarthritis can be caused by aging, heredity, and/or injury from trauma or disease. The <u>most common symptom of osteoarthritis is pain</u> in the affected joint(s). There is no blood test for the diagnosis of osteoarthritis. Repetitive use of the worn joints over the years can irritate and inflame the cartilage, causing joint pain and swelling. Loss of the cartilage cushion causes friction between the bones, leading to pain and limitation of joint mobility.

Inflammation of the cartilage can also stimulate new bone outgrowths (spurs, also referred to as osteophytes) to form around the joints. Osteoarthritis occasionally can develop in multiple members of the same family, implying a hereditary (genetic) basis for this condition. Secondary (type 2) osteoarthritis is a form of osteoarthritis that is caused by another disease or condition. Conditions that can lead to secondary osteoarthritis include obesity, repeated trauma to the joint structures, abnormal joints at birth (congenital abnormalities), gout, diabetes, and other hormone disorders.

Obesity causes osteoarthritis by increasing the mechanical stress on the joint and therefore on the cartilage. In fact, next to aging, obesity is the most significant risk factor for osteoarthritis of the knees. Crystal deposits in the cartilage can cause cartilage degeneration and osteoarthritis. Uric acid crystals cause gouty arthritis, while calcium pyrophosphate crystals cause arthritis in pseudo-gout. Some people are born with abnormally formed joints (congenital abnormalities) that are vulnerable to mechanical wear, causing early degeneration and loss of joint cartilage.

Osteoarthritis of the hip joints is commonly related to structural abnormalities of these joints that had been present since birth. Hormone disturbances, such as diabetes, thyroid and growth hormone disorders, are also associated with early cartilage wear and secondary osteoarthritis. Primary osteoarthritis is mostly a result of natural aging of the joint. With aging, the water content of the cartilage increases, and the protein makeup of cartilage degenerates. Eventually, cartilage begins to degenerate by flaking or forming tiny crevasses. In advanced osteoarthritis, there is a total loss of the cartilage cushion between the bones of the joints.

Symptoms and Signs: <u>The most common symptom of osteoarthritis is **pain** in the affected joint(s): especially after repetitive use</u>. Joint pain of osteoarthritis is usually worse later in the day. There can be swelling, warmth, and creaking of the affected joints. Pain and stiffness of the joints can also occur after long periods of inactivity (for example, sitting in a theater). In severe osteoarthritis, complete loss of the cartilage cushion causes friction between bones, causing pain even at rest or pain with limited motion.

Symptoms of osteoarthritis vary greatly from patient to patient. Some patients can be debilitated by their symptoms. On the other hand, others may have remarkably few symptoms in spite of dramatic degeneration of the joints apparent on X-rays. Symptoms also can be intermittent. It is not unusual for patients with osteoarthritis of the finger joints of the hands and knees to have years of pain-free intervals between symptoms.

Progressive cartilage degeneration of the knee joints can lead to deformity and outward curvature of the knees, which is referred to as being "bowlegged." People with osteoarthritis of the weight-bearing joints (such as the knees) can develop a limp. The limping can worsen as more cartilage degenerates. In some patients, the pain, limping, and joint dysfunction may not respond to medications or other conservative measures.

Therefore, severe osteoarthritis of the knees is one of the most common reasons for the <u>total knee replacement</u> -surgical procedures in the United States. Osteoarthritis of the cervical spine or lumbar spine causes pain in the neck or low back. Bony spurs, called osteophytes, that form along the arthritic spine can irritate spinal nerves, causing severe pain that can radiate from the spine as well as numbness and tingling of the affected parts of the body.

Osteoarthritis causes the formation of hard, bony enlargements of the small joints of the fingers. Classic boney enlargement of the small joint at the end of the fingers is called a <u>Heberden's node</u>, named after a famous British doctor. The bony deformity is a result of the <u>bone spurs</u> from the osteoarthritis in that joint. Another common bony knob (node) occurs at the middle joint of the fingers is called a <u>Bouchard's node</u>. Heberden's and Bouchard's nodes may not be painful, but they are often associated with limitation of motion of the joint. The characteristic appearances of these finger nodes can be helpful in diagnosing osteoarthritis.

Osteoarthritis of the joint at the base of the big toe of the foot leads to the formation of a <u>bunion</u>. Osteoarthritis of the fingers and the toes may have a genetic basis and can be found in numerous female members of some families. The prognosis of patients with osteoarthritis depends on which joints are affected and whether or not they are causing symptoms and impaired function. Some patients are unaffected by osteoarthritis while others can be severely disabled. Joint replacement surgery for some, results in the best long-term outcome. <u>Research scientists have found that doxycycline, a tetracycline drug, has been shown to slow the progression of cartilage degeneration in the knees of patients with osteoarthritis.</u> This effect seems to be a result of the drug's affect on enzymes that destroy cartilage rather than on their properties as antibiotics.

Nutritional Factors: Lifestyle and nutrition factors play an important role in both the prevention and treatment of osteoarthritis. Eating a balanced diet helps reduce inflammation and prevent obesity, a risk factor for osteoarthritis. Aim to eat plenty of fresh fruits and vegetables and avoid foods that contain trans-fatty acids such as margarine, shortening and products made with these hydrogenated oils, e.g., processed foods and cookies, etc. and even French fries. Choose lean meats such as fish and chicken over red meat and avoid refined foods.

Foods known to have anti-inflammatory properties include: <u>garlic, watercress, parsley, celery and cold-water fish</u>. Some supplements may also help to prevent the condition, especially omega 3 fish oils. Studies are underway to look at whether some glucosamine formulations may have advantages over others. The most common supplements used for joint health include glucosamine, chondroitin and (MSM) methylsulfonylmethane. Exercise with its anabolic effect, may at the same time stop or reverse osteoporosis. Medication includes calcium, vitamin D, bisphosphonates and several others.

PEPTIC ULCER DISEASE: A peptic ulcer, also known as PUD or peptic ulcer disease, is the most common ulcer of any acidic area of the gastrointestinal tract. It is usually extremely painful. It is defined as mucosal erosions equal to or greater than 0.5 cm. As many as 70–90% of such ulcers are associated with Helicobacter pylori, a spiral-shaped bacterium that lives in the acidic environment of the stomach. Ulcers can also be caused or worsened by drugs such as aspirin, ibuprofen, and other NSAIDs. Four times as many peptic ulcers arise in the duodenum, the first part of the small intestine just after the stomach, as in the stomach itself. About 4% of gastric (stomach) ulcers are caused by a malignant tumor, so multiple biopsies are needed to exclude cancer. Duodenal ulcers are generally benign.

Signs and symptoms: Symptoms of a peptic ulcer can be:

- abdominal pain, classically epigastric with severity relating to mealtimes, after around three hours of taking a meal (duodenal ulcers are classically relieved by food, while gastric ulcers are exacerbated by it):
- bloating and abdominal fullness:
- waterbrash (rush of saliva to dilute the acid:
- nausea and copious vomiting:

- loss of appetite and weight loss:
- hematemesis (vomiting of blood): this can occur due to bleeding directly from a gastric ulcer, or from damage to the esophagus from severe/continuing vomiting.
- melena (tarry, foul-smelling feces due to oxidized iron from hemoglobin).

Rarely, an ulcer can lead to a gastric or duodenal perforation, which would lead to acute peritonitis. This is extremely painful and requires immediate surgery. A history of heartburn, gastroesophageal reflux disease (GERD) and use of certain forms of medication can raise the suspicion for peptic ulcer. Medicines associated with peptic ulcer include NSAID (non-steroid anti-inflammatory drugs) that inhibit cyclooxygenase, and most steroids (e.g. dexamethasone and prednisolone). The timing of the symptoms in relation to the meal may differentiate between gastric and duodenal ulcers.

A gastric ulcer would give epigastric pain during the meal, as gastric acid production is increased as food enters the stomach. Symptoms of duodenal ulcers would initially be relieved by a meal, as the pyloric sphincter closes to concentrate the stomach contents, therefore acid is not reaching the duodenum.

Duodenal ulcer pain would manifest mostly 2–3 hours after the meal, when the stomach begins to release digested food and acid into the duodenum. The pain caused by peptic ulcers can be felt anywhere from the navel up to the sternum, it may last from few minutes to several hours and it may be worse when the stomach is empty.

Also, sometimes the pain may flare at night and it can commonly be temporarily relieved by eating foods that buffer stomach acid or by taking anti-acid medication. However, peptic ulcer disease symptoms may be different for every sufferer.

Causes: Peptic ulcers are open sores in the lining of the stomach, small intestine and/or esophagus caused by the bacteria Helicobacter pylori (H. pylori). Risk factors for peptic ulcers are heredity, age, a history of chronic pain, alcohol use, diabetes, stress and smoking. Symptoms include pain, burning, indigestion, gas, nausea, vomiting, weight loss and loss of appetite.

A major causative factor (60% of gastric and up to 90% of duodenal ulcers) is chronic inflammation due to Helicobacter pylori that colonizes the antral mucosa. The bacterium can cause a chronic active gastritis (type B gastritis), resulting in a defect in the regulation of gastrin production by that part of the stomach. Gastrin stimulates the production of gastric acid by parietal cells. In H. pylori colonization responses to increased gastrin, the increase in acid can contribute to the erosion of the mucosa and therefore ulcer formation.

Another major cause is the use of NSAIDs. The gastric mucosa protects itself from gastric acid with a layer of mucus, the secretion of which is stimulated by certain prostaglandins. NSAIDs block the function of cyclooxygenase 1 (cox-1), which is essential for the production of prostaglandins. Cox-2 selective anti-inflammatories (such as Celecoxib, Celebrex) inhibit Cox-2 and not Cox 1. Cox 2 is less essential in the gastric mucosa, and therefore Celebrex is able to relieve arthritis pain with roughly halve the risk of NSAID-related gastric ulceration.

The incidence of duodenal ulcers has dropped significantly during the last 30 years, while the incidence of gastric ulcers has shown a small increase, mainly caused by the widespread use of NSAIDs. Although some studies have found correlations between smoking and ulcer formation, others have been more specific in exploring the risks involved and have found that smoking by itself may not be much of a risk factor unless associated with H. pylori infection.

Some suggested risk factors such as diet, and spice consumption, were hypothesized as ulcerogens (helping cause ulcers) until late in the 20th century, but have been shown to be of relatively minor importance in the development of peptic ulcers. Gastrinomas (Zollinger Ellison syndrome), rare gastrin-secreting tumors, also cause multiple and difficult-to-heal ulcers.

Stress: Researchers also continue to look at stress as a possible cause, or at least complication, in the development of ulcers. Burns and head trauma can lead to physiologic stress ulcers, which are reported in many patients who are on mechanical ventilation. An expert panel concluded that ulcers are not always purely due to an infectious disease and that psychological factors do play a significant role. Some researchers are examining how stress might promote H. pylori infection. For example, Helicobacter pylori thrives in an acidic environment, and stress has been demonstrated to cause the production of excess stomach acid.

Nutritional factors: A special diet cannot prevent or cure an ulcer. However, certain foods (some listed below) may help relieve symptoms.

Fiber: Dietary fiber intake is associated with a decreased risk of developing peptic ulcers. A high-fiber diet is recommended for people with peptic ulcers because it speeds recovery. Fiber is in fruits, vegetables, beans, legumes and whole grains. In addition to easing peptic ulcer discomfort, fiber benefits heart health, stabilizes blood sugar and can help control weight.

Probiotics: Probiotics are live microorganisms that may benefit health. Studies show Long-term use of probiotics also lowered the risk of infection by H. pylori and development of peptic ulcers.

Common sources of probiotics are yogurt, miso, tempeh, some juices and soy beverages.

Flavonoids: Flavonoids are phytochemicals that are rich in antioxidants and have been linked to prevention of heart disease and cancer. Flavonoids function as antioxidants and have protective qualities that could be therapeutic in the treatment of peptic ulcers. Good sources of flavonoids that may inhibit bacterial growth are apples, celery, cranberries, onions, garlic and tea.

Low-Fat Foods: Many individuals with peptic ulcers also experience gastroesophageal reflux (GERD). According to the Mayo Clinic, controlling GERD is one way to minimize symptoms associated with a peptic ulcer. Fatty foods should be limited because they increase stomach acid, which can trigger GERD and irritate peptic ulcers. Decrease dietary fat by choosing lean meats, fruits, vegetables, whole grains, poultry, fish and low-fat dairy products.

PERIODONTAL DISEASE: Periodontitis is a set of inflammatory diseases affecting the periodontium, i.e., the tissues that surround and support the teeth. Periodontitis involves progressive loss of the alveolar bone around the teeth, and if left untreated, can lead to the loosening and subsequent loss of teeth.

Periodontitis is caused by microorganisms that adhere to and grow on the tooth's surfaces, along with an overly aggressive immune response against these microorganisms. A diagnosis of periodontitis is established by inspecting the soft gum tissues around the teeth with a probe (i.e., a clinical exam) and by evaluating the patient's x-ray films (radiographic exam), to determine the amount of bone loss around the teeth. Specialists in the treatment of periodontitis are periodontists: their field is known as "periodontology" or "periodontics".

Signs and Symptoms: In the early stages, periodontitis has very few symptoms and in many individuals the disease has progressed significantly before they seek treatment. Symptoms may include the following:

- ✓ Redness or bleeding of gums while brushing teeth, using dental floss or biting into hard food (e.g. apples) (though this may occur even in gingivitis, where there is no attachment loss)
- ✓ Gum swelling that recurs
- ✓ Spitting out blood after brushing teeth
- ✓ Halitosis, or bad breath, and a persistent metallic taste in the mouth
- ✓ Gingival recession, resulting in apparent lengthening of teeth. (This may also be caused by heavy handed brushing or with a stiff tooth brush.)
- ✓ Deep pockets between the teeth and the gums (pockets are sites where the attachment has been gradually destroyed by collagen-destroying enzymes)
- ✓ Loose teeth, in the later stages (though this may occur for other reasons as well).

Patients should realize that the gingival inflammation and bone destruction are largely painless. Hence, people may wrongly assume that painless bleeding after teeth cleaning is insignificant, although this may be a symptom of progressing periodontitis.

Effects outside the mouth: Periodontitis has been linked to increased inflammation in the body such as indicated by elevated levels of C-reactive protein (CRP) and elevated levels of Interleukin-6. It is through this link that there is an increased risk of stroke, myocardial infarction (heart attack), and atherosclerosis. It is also linked in those over 60 years of age to impairments in delayed memory and calculation abilities. Individuals with impaired fasting glucose and diabetes mellitus have higher degree of periodontal inflammation, and often have difficulties with balancing their blood glucose level owing to the constant systemic inflammatory state, caused by the periodontal inflammation.

Causes: Periodontitis is an inflammation of the periodontium, i.e., the tissues that support the teeth. The periodontium consists of four tissues: gingiva, or gum tissue: cementum, or outer layer of the roots of teeth: alveolar bone, or the bony sockets into which the teeth are anchored: periodontal ligaments (PDLs), which are the connective tissue fibers that run between the cementum and the alveolar bone.

Widening of the periodontal ligament surrounding the premolar is due to secondary occlusal trauma. The primary etiology (cause) of gingivitis is poor oral hygiene which leads to the accumulation of a mycotic and bacterial matrix at the gum line, called dental plaque. Other contributors are poor nutrition and underlying medical issues such as diabetes.

 If left undisturbed, microbic plaque calcifies to form calculus, which is commonly called tartar. Calculus above and below the gum line must be removed completely by the dental hygienist or dentist to treat gingivitis and periodontitis. Although the primary cause of both gingivitis and periodontitis is the microbic plaque that adheres to the tooth surface, there are many other modifying factors. A very strong risk factor is one's genetic susceptibility.

Several conditions and diseases, including Down syndrome, diabetes, candidiasis and other diseases that affect one's resistance to infection also increase susceptibility to periodontitis. Another factor that makes periodontitis a difficult disease to study is that human host response can also affect the alveolar bone resorption. Host response to the bacterial-mycotic insult is mainly determined by genetics: however, immune development may play some role in susceptibility. According to some researchers periodontitis may be associated with higher stress levels different individuals encounter.

Treatment:

Step 1: Brush your teeth at least twice daily. Be sure to brush both sides of your teeth in gentle circular motions. Brush your gums as well. The accumulation of plaque will only further compound the problem, so keep your teeth as clean as possible.

Step 2: Floss at least once daily: food has a tendency to lodge between teeth and further promotes the accumulation of plaque and bacteria that can weaken your gums. In dealing with periodontal disease, the importance of flossing cannot be expressed enough.

Step 3: Eat a balanced diet. If your immune system is healthy, it will be harder for bacteria to have an effect on you. Eat fruits, vegetables and whole grains while cutting back on unnecessary sugars that can negatively affect both your teeth and the rest of your overall health.

Step 4: Incorporate Listerine into your daily routine. An antiseptic mouthwash such as Listerine can help clean places that your toothbrush and sometimes even the floss can't: rinse twice daily with the Listerine for the best results.

Step 5: Schedule appointments with your dentist/periodontist and keep them. The fight against periodontal disease really needs to be fought on two fronts. The dentist can perform scaling and root planning to help clean under the gums and take a closer look at your progress. He can help to give you the right tips and advice in your own personal battle with periodontal disease.

Nutritional factors: Gingivitis is the first stage of gum disease, typically associated with red, swollen and bleeding gums. If left untreated, gingivitis can progress to a more advanced gum disease known as periodontitis. Regular dental checkups and cleaning is essential for the health of your gums. Your health care provider may recommend certain foods that can promote oral health and reduce your risk for gum disease.

Citrus Fruits: Citrus fruits are well known for their vibrant color, scent and taste. They include oranges, mandarins, tangerines, lemons, limes and grapefruits. Citrus fruits provide essential vitamins and are good sources of antioxidants, particularly vitamin C. Low intakes of vitamin C are linked to poor immune response. Individuals who are deficient of the vitamin are at greater risk for gum disease. Vitamin C found in citrus fruits can also promote tissue repair in the body and fight off infection.

Green Leafy Vegetables: Greens or leafy vegetables such as asparagus, broccoli, kale, cabbage, spinach and turnip greens are also part of a well-balanced diet. Similar to fruits, they provide beneficial vitamins and antioxidants, particularly vitamin E and folic acid. Individuals who are deficient of folic acid are more susceptible to harmful plaque that promote gum diseases. Green leafy vegetables are recommended for gum health because of their vitamin E content. Similar to vitamin C, vitamin E is a vitamin that has beneficial antioxidant abilities that protect cells from damage.

Fatty Fish: Fatty fish such as cod, salmon, tuna, trout, sardines and herring provide protein and essential fatty acids known as omega-3. One study observed the effects of omega-3 fatty acids on periodontitis. The study found that higher intakes of omega-3 fatty acids were associated with a reduced risk for gum disease. The protein found in fatty fish may also support immunity. Adequate intake of protein is necessary to support a healthy immune system and fight off infection.

<u>Nuts:</u> Nuts are packed with vitamins, minerals, fiber, protein and essential fatty acids. Some good examples of nuts include cashews, almonds and walnuts. **Zinc** is an essential mineral that is found in nuts. Individuals with zinc deficiencies are also more likely to suffer from bacteria that cause gum disease.

PROSTATE PROBLEMS: **Prostate Enlargement**: The prostate is a walnut-sized gland found only in men. It sits just below the bladder and surrounds the urethra, the tube that carries urine through the penis. The prostate's job is to make fluid for semen. The prostate grows naturally with age, usually without problems. For such a little gland, the prostate seems to cause a lot of concern.

 All men are at risk for prostate problems. <u>That's because all men have a prostate.</u> Benign prostatic hyperplasia (BPH). BPH, also known as an enlarged prostate, is growth of the prostate gland to an unhealthy size. A man's chances of having BPH go up with age: Take a look at this overview of prostate problems to assess your risk for trouble with your prostate.

age 31-40:	one in 12
age 51-60:	about one in two
over age 80:	more than eight in 10

However, only about one out of every two men ever has BPH symptoms that need treatment. <u>BPH does not lead to prostate cancer</u>, although both are common in older men and should be routinely tested for prostate cancer.

Prostate Cancer. Prostate cancer is the most common cancer in men (besides skin cancer). About one man in six will be diagnosed with prostate cancer in his lifetime. Let's keep these numbers in perspective, though. Because prostate cancer is usually slow growing, only about one in 35 men with prostate cancer will die of prostate cancer. Like BPH, the risk for prostate cancer increases with age. About two out of every three men with prostate cancer are over 65.

 No one knows exactly what causes prostate cancer, but risk factors associated with it include: (1) Family history. Having a father or brother with prostate cancer more than doubles your risk. (2) Race. African-American men are more likely to get prostate cancer than Caucasians, and the cancer is usually more advanced when discovered.

Prostate cancer often has no symptoms. It is often discovered after screening with a lab test called prostate specific antigen (PSA). Occasionally, prostate cancer can cause obstruction of urine flow, like BPH. This symptom usually suggests more advanced prostate cancer. Prostate cancer screening is controversial. Some doctors and organizations recommend regular screening while others don't. The discussion about screening should start at age 50 for most men with average risk for prostate cancer and earlier for men at higher risk. The American Urological Association recommends a first-time test at age 40, with the schedule of follow-up testing to be determined on an individual basis.

Prostatitis. On the scientific level, the causes of prostatitis are not completely understood. There is controversy among the most highly regarded experts. Keep in mind that any one patient may have more than one cause operating at the same time. There are three main schools of thought about the causes of prostatitis. Bacterial infection, Auto-immune response or disordered immune response, Neuromuscular, tension or physical injury problem.

Additional possible causes: a uric acid disorder, prostate stones, a urethral stricture, a rare tumor, prostate cancer, benign prostatic hyperplasia (BPH, non-cancerous growth of the prostate), a food allergy, a yeast infestation, a specific yeast problem from the

Genus Candida, or a virus. Unlike most prostate problems, prostatitis, inflammation or an infection of the prostate, occurs more often in young and middle-aged men. Only 5% to 10% of men develop prostatitis in their lifetime. Think of prostatitis as a type of men's urinary tract infection. Possible symptoms include: pain on urinating or ejaculating, fever and chills, pelvic pain, needing to urinate more often, cloudy urine. Prostate infection is rarely serious, but if you have symptoms of prostatitis, see your doctor. Prostatitis is most often treated with antibiotics, usually for at least four weeks.

Treatment depends on which kind of prostate problem you develop.

In some ways, prostate problems, particularly BPH, are a natural part of growing older. Still, there are specific steps you can take to keep your prostate healthy.

- A diet low in saturated fat and high in fruits and vegetables may lower your risk of developing BPH.
- No herbal supplements have been proven to prevent prostate cancer. Studies of selenium, a mineral that has shown some promise, are underway. Trials for drugs to prevent prostate cancer are also ongoing.
- No activity or drug is known to prevent prostatitis.
- Experts recommend good hygiene, including keeping the penis clean.

Most men will never develop prostatitis.

Only about one out of every two men ever has BPH symptoms that need treatment. BPH does not lead to prostate cancer, although both are common in older men.

<u>Benign prostatic hyperplasia (BPH) needs treatment only if the urinary symptoms become bothersome.</u> BPH often responds to drugs that either:

> (A) relieve the tension around the urethra (Cardura, Flomax, Hytrin, and Uroxatral)

> (B) reduce the size of the prostate itself (Avodart and Proscar)

The FDA is revising labels on several BPH drugs -- Proscar, Avodart, and Jalyn -- to include a warning that the drugs may be linked to an increased risk of prostate cancer. If medication does not relieve the symptoms, surgery may be required.

Prostate cancer treatment is complex. When designing a prostate cancer treatment plan, doctors consider a man's age, overall health, and how aggressive or widely spread the prostate cancer is. Each man's cancer is unique, and his treatment will be unique. Some treatment options include: no treatment (watchful waiting), surgery, radiation (either external-beam or implantable "seeds"), chemotherapy, a combination of these.

Nutritional factors: Several herbs showed promise as treatment for BPH in some studies, but results are incomplete or conflicting. These include saw palmetto, beta-sitosterol, Selenium and zinc and Pygeum africanum.

<u>Best Foods:</u> Figs are known as one of the best fruits for the prostate health as well as for the testicles. Some of the best foods are those with the highest levels of **selenium and zinc** which

include: shellfish, especially oysters, certain grains, wheat germ and wheat bran. All-bran cereal is also a good choice. If you like beer, you're in luck--brewer's yeast has high levels of zinc, with as much per 100 g as wheat germ. All nuts and seed but especially Pine nuts and pecans are also good choices. Many protein-rich foods are also rich in selenium and zinc, including ham, beef and lamb. Note: Vitamin E, vitamin C, beta-carotene, selenium and zinc are common antioxidants found in fruits and vegetables that are especially good for prostate health. Colorful fruits and vegetables contain the highest levels of these antioxidants, especially those that are purple, blue, red, orange and yellow and dark leafy greens.

OK Foods: If none of the foods above appeal to you, or if you need additional choices, some foods have lower but still adequate levels of selenium and zinc. For example, Liver, Cashew nuts, Parmesan cheese. If you do not like shellfish, try regular fish. Eggs are also a decent source, especially considering that the average person probably eats more eggs than cashew nuts, fish or liver.

Things to Avoid: Multivitamins containing selenium and zinc might sound like a great idea, but because the zinc compounds in the multivitamins are inorganic, they are actually much harder for your body to absorb, and the zinc that you take in can pass directly through your body without actually helping you with your prostate problems. If you are taking a calcium or iron supplement, or have a large amount of copper in your bloodstream, speak with your doctor to find out if they will inhibit zinc absorption. You should also avoid foods that make your prostate or bladder problems worse. Caffeinated drinks can be bad for an enlarged prostate. Spread your liquid consumption throughout the day, and avoid drinking two hours before bed.

PSORIASIS: Psoriasis is an autoimmune disease that affects the skin. It occurs when the immune system mistakes the skin cells as a pathogen, and sends out faulty signals that speed up the growth cycle of skin cells. Psoriasis is not contagious. There are five types of psoriasis: plaque, guttate, inverse, pustular, and erythrodermic. The most common form, plaque psoriasis, is commonly seen as red and white hues of scaly patches appearing on the top first layer of the epidermis (skin). Some patients, though, have no dermatological signs or symptoms. In plaque psoriasis, skin rapidly accumulates at these sites, which gives it a silvery-white appearance. Plaques frequently occur on the skin of the elbows and knees, but can affect any area, including the scalp, palms of hands and soles of feet, and genitals.

 In contrast to eczema, psoriasis is more likely to be found on the outer side of the joint. The disorder is a chronic recurring condition that varies in severity from minor localized patches to complete body coverage. Fingernails and toenails are frequently affected (psoriatic nail dystrophy) and can be seen as an isolated sign. Psoriasis can also cause inflammation of the joints, which is known as psoriatic arthritis. Between 10—30% of all people with psoriasis also have psoriatic arthritis. The cause of psoriasis is not fully understood, but it is believed to have a genetic component that is triggered by an injury to the skin known as the Koebner phenomenon. Various environmental factors have been suggested as aggravating to psoriasis, including stress, withdrawal of systemic corticosteroid, as well as other environmental factors, but few have shown statistical significance.

Signs and Symptoms: Quality of life. Severe cases of psoriasis have been shown to affect health-related quality of life to an extent similar to the effects of other chronic diseases, such as depression, hypertension, congestive heart failure and/or type 2 diabetes. Depending on the severity and location of outbreaks, individuals may experience significant physical discomfort and some disability. Itching and pain can interfere with basic functions, such as self-care, walking, and sleep. Plaques on hands and feet can prevent individuals from working at certain occupations, playing some sports, and caring for family members or a home. Plaques on the scalp can be particularly embarrassing, as flaky plaque in the hair can be mistaken for dandruff. Medical care can be costly and time-consuming, and can interfere with an employment or school schedule. Individuals with psoriasis may also feel self-conscious about their appearance and have a poor self-image that stems from fear of public rejection and psychosexual concerns. Psychological distress can lead to significant depression and social isolation. More than half of those diagnosed with psoriasis reported significant feelings of self-consciousness and embarrassment. More than one-third said they avoided social activities and limited dating or intimate interactions.

Causes: The cause of psoriasis is not fully understood. There are two main hypotheses about the process that occurs in the development of the disease.

The <u>first</u> considers psoriasis as primarily a disorder of excessive growth and reproduction of skin cells. The problem is simply seen as a fault of the epidermis and its keratinocytes.

The <u>second</u> hypothesis sees the disease as being an immune-mediated disorder in which the excessive reproduction of skin cells is secondary to factors produced by the immune system. T cells (which normally help protect the body against infection) become active, migrate to the dermis and trigger the release of cytokines (tumor necrosis factor-alpha TNFα, in particular) which cause inflammation and the rapid production of skin cells.

It is not known what initiates the activation of the T cells. The immune-mediated model of psoriasis has been supported by the observation that immunosuppressant medications can clear psoriasis plaques. Compromised skin barrier function has a role in psoriasis susceptibility. Psoriasis is a fairly an idiosyncratic disease. The majority of people's experience of psoriasis is one in which it may worsen or improve for no apparent reason. The first outbreak is sometimes reported following stress (physical and mental), skin injury, and streptococcal infection. Conditions that have been reported as accompanying a worsening of the disease include infections, stress, and changes in season and climate.

Certain medicines, including lithium salt, beta blockers and the anti-malarial drug chloroquine have been reported to trigger or aggravate the disease. Excessive alcohol consumption, smoking and obesity may exacerbate psoriasis or make the management of the condition difficult or perhaps these co-morbidities are effects rather than causes. Hairspray, some face creams and hand lotions, can also cause an outbreak of psoriasis.

 It is important to remember that most individuals with psoriasis are otherwise healthy. Psoriasis occurs more likely in dry skin than oily or well-moisturized skin, and specifically after an external skin injury such as a scratch or cut. This is believed to be caused by an infection, in which the infecting organism thrives under dry skin conditions with minimal skin oil, which otherwise protects skin from infections. The case for psoriasis is opposite to the case of athlete's foot, which occurs because of a fungus infection under wet conditions as opposed to dry conditions in psoriasis. This infection induces inflammation, which causes the symptoms commonly associated with psoriasis, such as itching and rapid skin turnover, and leads to drier skin, as the infecting organism absorbs the moisture that would otherwise go to the skin. To prevent dry skin and reduce psoriasis symptoms, it is advised to not use shower scrubs, as they not only damage skin by leaving tiny scratches, but they also scrape off the naturally occurring skin oil. Additionally, moisturizers can be applied to moisturize the skin, and lotions used to promote skin oil gland functions.

Management: There are a number of different treatment options for psoriasis. Typically, topical agents are used for mild disease, phototherapy for moderate disease, and systemic agents for severe disease. Topical agents: Bath solutions and moisturizers, mineral oil, and petroleum jelly may help soothe affected skin and reduce the dryness which accompanies the build-up of skin on psoriatic plaques.

Medicated creams and ointments applied directly to psoriatic plaques can help reduce inflammation, remove built-up scale, reduce skin turn over, and clear affected skin of plaques. Ointment and creams containing coal tar, dithranol (anthralin), corticosteroids, i.e., desoximetasone (Topicort), fluocinonide, vitamin D3 analogues (i.e., calcipotriol), and retinoids are routinely used. The mechanism of action of each is probably different, but they all help to normalize skin cell production and reduce inflammation. Activated vitamin D and its analogues can inhibit skin cell proliferation.

Phototherapy: in the form of sunlight has long been used effectively for treatment. Wavelengths of 311–313 nm are most effective and special lamps have been developed for this application. The exposure time should be controlled to avoid over exposure and burning of the skin. The UVB lamps should have a timer that will turn off the lamp when the time ends. The amount of light used is determined by a person's skin type. Psoralen and ultraviolet A phototherapy (PUVA) combines the oral or topical administration of psoralen with exposure to ultraviolet A (UVA) light. PUVA is associated with nausea, headache, fatigue, burning, and itching. Long-term treatment is associated with squamous cell carcinoma (but not with melanoma).

Systemic agents: Psoriasis that is resistant to topical treatment and phototherapy is treated by medications taken internally by pill or injection (systemic). Patients undergoing systemic treatment are required to have regular blood and liver function tests because of the toxicity of the medication. Pregnancy must be avoided for the majority of these treatments. Most people experience a recurrence of psoriasis after systemic treatment is discontinued. The three main traditional systemic treatments are methotrexate, cyclosporine and retinoids.

Methotrexate and cyclosporine are immunosuppressant drugs: retinoids are synthetic forms of the vitamin A. Biologics are usually given by self-injection or in a doctor's office. Two drugs that target T cells are efalizumab (Amevive) and alefacept (Raptiva). Efalizumab is a monoclonal anti-body which blocks the molecules that dendritic cells use to communicate with T cells. It also blocks the adhesion molecules on the endothelial cells that line blood vessels, which attract T cells. However, it suppressed the immune system's ability to control normally harmless viruses, which led to fatal brain infections. Alefacept also blocks the molecules that dendritic cells use to communicate with T cells. The psoriasis treatment ladder. As a first step, medicated ointments or creams, called topical treatments, are applied to the skin. If topical treatment fails to achieve the desired goal, then the next step would be to expose the skin to ultraviolet (UV) radiation. This type of treatment is called phototherapy. The third step involves the use of medications which are taken internally by pill or injection. This approach is called systemic treatment. The combination therapy for moderate to severe psoriasis using psoralen with ultraviolet A (PUVA) plus acitretin shows a 97.3% improvement from baseline.

Nutritional factors: Some studies suggest psoriasis symptoms can be relieved by changes in diet and lifestyle. Detoxification, periods of fasting, low energy diets and vegetarian diets have improved psoriasis symptoms in some patients, and diets supplemented with fish oil (e.g. cod liver oil) have also shown beneficial effects. Fish oils are rich in the two omega-3 fatty acids (EPA) eicosapentaenoic acid, (DHA) docosahexaenoic acid and Vitamin E, furthermore cod liver oil besides containing omega-3-fatty acids also contains

Vitamin A and Vitamin D. The following is a list of some very <u>good</u> <u>anti-psoriasis foods</u> that can help fight this unpleasant condition. Start eating these foods on a regular basis!

#1: Salmon: Salmon provides an excellent source of omega 3-fatty acids which have strong anti-inflammatory properties. Salmon also contains astaxanthin, a carotenoid that gives salmon its pink color and that can act as a potent antioxidant. The FDA recommends eating fish twice a week.

#2: Turmeric: Due to the wide-range of health benefits, turmeric has been used in Chinese and Ayurvedic medicine for centuries. It is known for its anti-inflammatory properties, and anecdotal evidence indicates that this powerful root plant of the ginger family may also be able to fend of psoriasis symptoms. Turmeric is a key ingredient in Indian style curries, but its range of culinary uses is in fact much wider. It can be used to add flavor to fish, seafood, meat, rice, vegetable, and pasta dishes. It is the main spice in mustard.

#3: Garlic: Few foods are better than garlic when it comes to healing disease and promoting health. Since prehistoric times, this magical medicinal plant has been used to treat and cure a wide range of health problems in humans. Recent research has shown it to be effective at controlling hypertension, preventing heart disease, preventing and treating cancer, and many infections: e.g., bacterial, viral, and/or fungal . Garlic can inhibit the activity of enzymes that generate inflammatory substances responsible for psoriasis symptoms.   Eating garlic on a daily basis may also be helpful for psoriasis patients. The beneficial effects of garlic on psoriasis are due to garlic's ability to inhibit the activity of lipoxygenase, an enzyme that is involved in the inflammatory cascade caused by arachidonic acid. Proriasis patients typically have high levels of arachidonic acid in their skin and fatty tissues. In addition, garlic—especially fresh garlic—contains a fair amount of vitamin C. It is also a good source of the antioxidant.

#4: Lettuce: Many naturopaths advocate the consumption of lettuce to combat psoriasis symptoms. Lettuce is thought to help improve digestion and promote liver health. It also provides a concentrated source of beta-carotene and a good source of vitamin C and folate. When buying lettuce, it is advisable to choose organically grown produce whenever possible.

#5: Broccoli: is chock-full of antioxidants and folate. Broccoli is inarguably one of the best foods for people with psoriasis as it is packed with beta-carotene, vitamin C, and folate. It also ranks low on the glycemic index. To get the most out of broccoli's health benefits, choose organically grown plants (they are typically more nutrient-dense and contain fewer harmful substances) and eat them raw or slightly steamed.

#6: Carrots: Most people know that carrots are good for our eyes, but most do not know that they can also be helpful for people suffering from psoriasis. Carrots are one of the best dietary sources of beta-carotene, but that's not all: they also contain vitamin C and a wealth of other nutrients.

#7: Fish Eggs are loaded with anti- inflammatory omega-3 fatty acids such as DHA and EPA. Fish eggs, one of the best natural sources of DHA and EPA. DHA and EPA are types omega-3 fatty acids which, due to their strong anti-inflammatory properties, may help prevent and manage psoriasis breakouts. Ounce for ounce, fish eggs contain even more omega-3's than the fattiest fish.

#8: Sweet Potatoes: which have been consumed since prehistoric times, are one of the most nutritious vegetables and an excellent addition to your diet if you suffer from psoriasis. They are among the foods that are least likely to cause allergic reactions, which is great news since psoriasis is often linked to allergies. The pink, orange, and yellow varieties are one of the most concentrated food sources of beta-carotene (the more intense the color, the more beta-carotene). Sweet potatoes also boast vitamin C, and they have a surprisingly low glycemic rating.

#9: Chicory Greens: The bitter-tasting leaves of the chicory plant are a very good source of beta-carotene and folate. They also contain vitamin C and vitamin E, both of which are potent antioxidants. In addition, chicory greens are low in calories, making them an attractive food also for dieters. Chicory greens can be eaten raw or cooked.

#10: Turnip Greens: Turnip greens, the leaves of the an ancient vegetable that was cultivated in the Near East already 4,000 years ago, are chock-full of important psoriasis-fighting nutrients including beta-carotene, vitamin C, and folate. Turnip is a member of the Brassica genus of plants, which comprises many other health-promoting plants such as cabbage, broccoli, and collards.

#11: Buckwheat: Despite its name, buckwheat is not related to wheat and does not contain gluten, which makes it a great alternative to wheat and many other grains for people whose psoriasis is linked to a gluten allergy. Buckwheat groats contain only 92 calories per 100 grams, which is also great news since a low calorie diet has been shown to improve the skin in psoriasis patients.

Additionally, buckwheat groats are packed with high quality protein, making it an excellent food for those who are watching their waistline.

The severity of psoriasis symptoms may also be influenced by lifestyle habits related to alcohol, smoking, weight, sleep, stress and exercise. It has been suggested that cannabis might treat psoriasis, due to the anti-inflammatory properties of its cannabinoids, and their regulatory effects on the immune system. The adverse effects of cannabis might be avoided with a topical preparation or by the use of (a) more specific endo-cannabinoid receptor agonist(s).

CARLA D. O. SHARBONO, M.D.

RHEUMATOID ARTHRITIS: Rheumatoid arthritis (RA) is a chronic, systemic inflammatory disorder that may affect many tissues and organs, but principally attacks flexible (synovial) joints. The process involves an inflammatory response of the capsule around the joints (synovium) secondary to swelling (hyperplasia) of synovial cells, excess synovial fluid, and the development of fibrous tissue (pannus) in the synovium. Pannus is the main feature that separates RA from osteoarthritis.

Signs and Symptoms: The pathology of the disease process often leads to the destruction of articular cartilage and ankylosis (fusion) of the joints. Rheumatoid arthritis, itself, can also produce diffuse inflammation in the lungs, membrane around the heart (pericardium), and white of the eye (sclera), and also nodular lesions, most common in subcutaneous tissue.

Also, autoimmunity plays a pivotal role in both its chronicity and progression. RA is considered a systemic autoimmune disease. It can be a very disabling and painful condition, which can lead to substantial loss of functioning, mobility and even loss of life if not adequately treated. It is a clinical diagnosis made on the basis of symptoms, physical exam, radiographs (X-rays) and labs. Diagnosis and long-term management are typically performed by a rheumatologist, an expert in joint, muscle and bone diseases.

Various treatments are available. Non-pharmacological treatment includes physical therapy, orthoses, occupational therapy and nutritional therapy but these do not stop the progression of joint destruction. Analgesia (painkillers) and anti-inflammatory drugs, including steroids, are used to suppress the symptoms, while disease-modifying anti-rheumatic drugs (DMARDs) are required to inhibit or halt the underlying immune process.

Nutritional factors: Clinical trials have shown that consumption of fish oil reduces the number of swollen joints for people with

226

rheumatoid arthritis and provides a beneficial anti-inflammatory effect. It also provides a protective effect for occlusive cardiovascular disease, for which people with RA are at risk. Some supplements may also help to prevent the condition altogether: although scientific evidence to prove this is limited. Eating a balanced diet helps reduce inflammation and prevent obesity. Aim to eat plenty of fresh fruits and vegetables and <u>avoid foods that contain trans-fatty acids</u> and high glycemic carbohydrates, such as candies and cookies, etc. Choose fish and chicken over red meat and avoid refined processed foods. Foods known to have anti-inflammatory properties, which include garlic, watercress, parsley, celery and cold-water fish, also help reduce pain, and swelling as well as progression of the disease. Actually these foods are good for any skin or joint disorder.

SEXUAL DISORDERS: **(FEMALE AND MALE)** The term "sexual dysfunction" is an umbrella term covering disorders that include male impotence, erectile dysfunction, premature ejaculation, problems with libido, vaginal spasms, painful intercourse and other problems that interfere with sexual desire and pleasure. While many people accept that diminished libido, impotence and physical symptoms, i.e., vaginal dryness, come along with age, there's a great deal of **evidence that nutrition and health have far more of an effect on maintaining healthy sexual functioning than the medical world once believed.** Research has established that, the overwhelming majority of cases of sexual dysfunction have a root physical cause that can be treated, and often treated easily. Sexual dysfunction is also far more common than most people know. There are varying reports that suggest sexual dysfunction may affect as much as 51% of men and 63% of women in the United States. Because many people are uncomfortable discussing such a private aspect of their lives with their doctors, many medical authorities feel that the incidence of sexual dysfunction is vastly under-reported.

What Sexual Dysfunction Does: Sexual well-being is a large part of most people's identity. When something affects the ability to become or remain aroused, to enjoy sexual activity and intimacy or to achieve orgasm, there can be a ripple effect that touches on family relationships, partner relationships and even job performance. Sexual dysfunction can become a factor in depression, and contribute to feelings of inadequacy and worthlessness.

Symptoms of Sexual Dysfunction:

Male Sexual Dysfunction

1. Impotence (erectile dysfunction). Impotence is defined as difficulty achieving or maintaining erection.
2. Premature ejaculation: The definitions for premature ejaculation vary widely, but the common denominator is that premature ejaculation is "persistent or recurrent ejaculation with minimal sexual stimulation."
3. Diminished libido is characterized by a lack of sexual desire.

Female Sexual Dysfunction

1. Dysfunction Vaginismus: Involuntary spasms of the vagina that make intercourse painful.
2. Dyspareunia
3. Persistent or recurrent genital pain that accompanies sexual intercourse
4. Vaginal dryness can contribute to painful intercourse. It may be due to lack of arousal, or to an underlying

physical cause such as low levels of needed hormones to produce sufficient lubrication.

Sexual Dysfunction that applies to both sexes

1. Sexual arousal disorder is defined as the inability to become or remain aroused despite adequate physical stimulation
2. Orgasmic disorder is the inability to reach orgasm despite arousal and sufficient sexual stimulation.

What Causes Sexual Dysfunction:

There are many causes for sexual dysfunction. Because sexual well-being is so intimately involved with personal identity and happiness, what begins as a physical reaction to a lack in the body can become a self-perpetuating problem as stress and anxiety create more pressure to overcome the problem. Some of the most common causes of sexual dysfunctions include:

Physical Illness or Systemic Conditions: Hypertension, diabetes and heart conditions can all contribute to sexual dysfunction. Circulatory disorders, or any condition that affects the circulation can prevent blood flow to the sexual organs – one of the prime ingredients of sexual arousal for both men and women.

Side effects of medications: Many widely prescribed medications for treatment of depression and hypertension can lower the libido and decrease sexual desire. In addition, SSRIs can depress the release of serotonin and other chemicals that contribute to arousal and orgasm.

Low levels of nitric acid in the blood: Associated with high blood pressure, low levels of nitric acid in the blood can also contribute to both erectile dysfunction in men and arousal dysfunction in women.

Depression or mood disorders: One of the major symptoms of depression is a lack of sexual desire or interest. While depression was once believed to have a purely psychological origin, medical evidence has proved that the majority of cases of depression have physical causes – most notably, <u>a lack of vitamin B</u> and <u>a deficiency of essential fatty acids</u> that are vital for the synthesis of enzymes and hormones necessary for maintaining healthy neural systems.

Treatments for Sexual Dysfunction: The treatment for sexual dysfunction is dependent on the cause, but there are some basic self-help strategies that have been shown to be effective.

Reduce Stress: Stress is more than just an emotional problem. It makes demands on the body's reserves of essential nutrients. Keeping those stores of nutrients replenished is a big step toward avoiding the physical effects of stress. In particular, research has shown that the B vitamins, folic acid (folate), vitamin B12 and omega 3 essential fatty acids found in fish oil can help relieve stress and treat many other causes of sexual dysfunction.

Nutritional Factors: As you age, testosterone levels begin to decline. Although taking testosterone supplements are an option, increasing certain foods in your diet might help improve testosterone levels.

* Cruciferous Vegetables: Eating more cruciferous vegetables, such as cabbage, cauliflower and broccoli, might boost testosterone production in the body by getting rid of excess estrogen. Too much estrogen in the body diminishes testosterone output. Scientists from the Rockefeller University Hospital and the University of Helsinki in Finland observed that the compound indole-3-carbinol, which is found in cruciferous vegetables, increases urinary output of estrogen in men.

* Garlic: Increasing your intake of garlic might increase testosterone levels, according to a study performed by researchers from Kobe's Women's University in Japan. They observed that rats following a high-protein diet with garlic powder for 28 days experienced increases in testosterone compared with those adhering to the same diet without garlic powder. Garlic contains the compound diallyldisulfide, which enhances the release of a hormone that stimulates testosterone production.

* Sweet Potatoes - Although vitamin A is most notably associated with eyesight, it may also play a role in testosterone output. According to research published in the June 2004 issue of "Clinical Endocrinology," researchers from the Kaplan Medical Center in Israel found that boys with delayed puberty <u>consuming vitamin A supplementation for six months experience significant increases in testosterone</u>. Sweet potatoes, carrots, eggs, squash and cantaloupe are good sources of vitamin A.

* Mushrooms - Vitamin D, which is found in dairy products, salmon, eggs and mushrooms, may improve testosterone levels.

Eat a healthy diet with less sugar and processed meats as well as hydrogenated oils. Because so many of the conditions associated with sexual dysfunction are affected by diet, maintaining a healthy diet that provides all the essential nutrients for health is a key element in maintaining healthy sexual functioning. Although fruits may not conjure the same images of manliness associated with steak and other hearty foods, **some fruits may help to increase your levels of testosterone, the primary male sex hormone. Testosterone helps both male and females to enhance muscle mass and reduce body fat, so you may find fruits beneficial for improving your body composition.**

* Bananas - are rich in complex carbohydrates, which can make them helpful for fueling workouts or daily activities. Carbohydrates

CARLA D. O. SHARBONO, M.D.

are also important for maintaining your testosterone levels if you're involved in athletic training. A study from the April 2010 edition of "European Journal of Applied Physiology" found that consuming a larger amount carbohydrates after exercise corresponded to an increase in testosterone levels.

* **Raisins** - Like bananas, raisin are also rich in carbohydrates. Additionally, one cup of raisins provides 12 percent of the daily suggested intake of magnesium, a mineral that helps to manage blood sugar levels and normal nerve and muscle function and can increase testosterone levels.

***Dried Figs**.- Dried figs are beneficial because they are rich in carbohydrates and provide 15 g of fiber per cup. Additionally, one cup of dried figs contains 24 percent of the daily suggested intake of calcium, a nutrient that supports strong bones and teeth and promotes higher testosterone levels.

***Avocado** - Avocados are a distinctive fruit due to their rough black skin and bright green pulp. Avocados also differ from many other fruits because they are high in fat (good fats):

* **Watermelon, cantaloupe, and cucumbers** - contain a large amount of L-arginine the amino acid responsible for making nitric acid, the main component of Viagra and Cialis.

Consuming more healthy dietary fat can increase your levels of testosterone. Because so many of the conditions associated with sexual dysfunction are affected by diet, maintaining a healthy diet that provides all the essential nutrients for health is a key element in maintaining healthy sexual functioning. Besides these common sense strategies, there are a number of herbs and supplements that have proven effective in treating diminished libido and other sexual dysfunctions.

232

*L-arginine - Because L-arginine is a <u>precursor to nitric acid</u>, which <u>promotes circulation of blood</u>, it can increase the blood flow to the genitals that is necessary for physical arousal. In one study, women given a multi-vitamin supplement that contained L-arginine reported approximately 40% greater improvement in achieving arousal and orgasm than those given a placebo. Studies with men have shown similar improvement in erectile dysfunction.

*Ginkgo biloba - has been used in traditional medicine for centuries to restore energy and increase sexual libido. Several small studies have shown positive results with depression-induced sexual dysfunction.

*DHEA - is a naturally occurring hormone that is converted in the body to both testosterone and estrogen. Because one of the primary causes of vaginal dryness and tissue problems in post-menopausal women is lack of estrogen, DHEA can help relieve painful intercourse and stimulate the body to produce more natural lubricants.

Because the causes of sexual dysfunction are many, there is no one surefire cure-all. There is, however, a lot of evidence to support the importance of maintaining overall health with regular activity and high quality nutrition. Because it's difficult to get all the nutrients your body needs every single day, a high quality nutritional supplement can be a valuable ally in your quest for overall health.

THYROID PROBLEMS: The thyroid gland produces hormones that play an important role in your metabolism, energy, mood and overall health.

Signs and Symptoms: If you have <u>hypothyroidism</u>, meaning your thyroid produces too few hormones, you may experience lethargy, depressed moods (depression), weight gain, constipation, high cholesterol and menstrual problems. An overactive thyroid is <u>hyperthyroidism</u>: it causes opposing symptoms, such as a rapid heartbeat, anxiety, insomnia and weight loss. In addition to medical treatments, when necessary, your diet may play a valuable role in managing your symptoms.

Nutritional Info: While dietary changes are not known to cure thyroid conditions, they may prevent and aid in the treatment thus reducing your symptoms. In mild cases, improving your glycemic load, or the impact your diet has on your blood sugar, may help restore proper thyroid levels. Dietary changes may also help reverse or prevent complications of thyroid diseases, such as unintentional weight gain or loss.

Helpful Foods: To manage side effect of both thyroid problems, i.e., constipation, blood sugar imbalances and increased appetite consume fiber-rich foods such as whole grain breads, brown rice, pearled barley and legumes as well as most vegetables and fruits: especially antioxidant-rich foods such as berries, citrus fruits, bell peppers and winter squash. These foods help reduce symptoms of hypothyroidism and hyperthyroidism. Antioxidants such as vitamin C and beta-carotene also strengthen your body's ability to fend off additional health problems. For reduced inflammation and improved immune function and heart health, routinely incorporate omega-3 fatty acid sources such as salmon, herring, mackerel, fish oil, flaxseed, walnuts and canola oil, into your diet routinely.

Foods to Limit: Limit refined foods such as enriched breads, candy and potato chips which may offset your blood sugar and energy levels and leave less room for nutritious food. If you have hyperthyroidism, eliminate suspected food allergens such as dairy products, wheat, corn, soy, and especially chemical food additives and preservatives. If your thyroid is underactive, limit foods that may interfere with thyroid function such as broccoli, cauliflower, cabbage, Brussels sprout, leafy greens, millet, pine nuts, peanuts, turnips and soybeans.

  Avoid fatty, red and processed meats as well as butter, hard margarine and shortening, which may increase inflammation and damage your cholesterol levels and heart health. To reduce anxiety, insomnia and rapid heartbeat, limit caffeine and other stimulants, such as ginseng, caffeinated teas and regular soft drinks, particularly near bedtime. For example, consume oatmeal, low-fat yogurt, fresh fruit and flaxseed for breakfast, and brown rice, salmon and vegetables for lunch.

URINARY TRACT INFECTION: A urinary tract infection (UTI) is a bacterial infection that affects part of the urinary tract. When it affects the lower urinary tract it is known as a simple <u>cystitis</u> (a bladder infection) and when it affects the upper urinary tract it is known as <u>pyelonephritis</u> (a kidney infection).

Signs and Symptoms and Causes: Symptoms from a lower urinary tract infection include: painful urination and either frequent urination or urge to urinate (or both), while those of pyelonephritis include fever and flank pain in addition to the symptoms of a lower UTI. In the elderly and the very young, symptoms may be vague or non specific, e.g., tired, lethargy, confusion, irritability.

Cause: The main causal agent of both types is Escherichia coli, however other bacteria, viruses or fungi may rarely be the cause. Urinary tract infections occur more commonly in women than men, with half of the women having at least one infection at some point in their lives. Recurrences are common. Risk factors include female anatomy, sexual intercourse and family history.

Pyelonephritis, if it occurs, usually follows a bladder infection but may also result from a blood borne infection. Diagnosis in young healthy women can be based on symptoms alone. In those with vague symptoms, diagnosis can be difficult because bacteria may be present without there being an infection. In complicated cases or if treatment has failed, a urine culture may be useful. In those with frequent infections, low dose antibiotics may be taken as a preventative measure. In uncomplicated cases, urinary tract infections are easily treated with a short course of antibiotics, although resistance to many of the antibiotics used to treat this condition is increasing.

In complicated cases, a longer course or intravenous antibiotics may be needed, and if symptoms have not improved in two or three days, further diagnostic testing is needed. In women, urinary tract infections are the most common form of bacterial infection with 10% developing urinary tract infections yearly.

Urine may contain pus (a condition known as <u>pyuria</u>) as seen from a person with <u>sepsis</u> due to a urinary tract infection. Lower urinary tract infection is also referred to as a bladder infection. The most common symptoms are <u>burning with urination</u> and having to urinate frequently (or an urge to urinate) in the absence of <u>vaginal discharge</u> and significant pain. These symptoms may vary from mild to severe and in healthy women last an average of six days. Some pain above the <u>pubic bone</u> or in the <u>lower back</u> may be present.

People experiencing an upper urinary tract infection, or <u>pyelonephritis</u>, may experience <u>flank pain</u>, <u>fever</u>, or nausea and <u>vomiting</u> in addition to the classic symptoms of a lower urinary tract infection. Rarely the urine may appear bloody or contain visible <u>pyuria</u> (pus in the urine). In young children, the only symptom of a urinary tract infection (UTI) may be a fever. Because of the lack of more obvious symptoms, when females under the age of two or uncircumcised males less than a year exhibit a fever, a culture of the urine is recommended by many medical associations.

Infants may feed poorly, vomit, sleep more, or show signs of <u>jaundice</u>. In older children, new onset <u>urinary incontinence</u> (loss of bladder control) may occur. In the elderly, urinary tract symptoms are frequently lacking. The presentations may be vague with incontinence, a <u>change in mental status</u>, or fatigue as the only symptoms. While some present to a health care provider with <u>sepsis</u>, an infection of the blood, as the first symptoms.

Diagnosis can be complicated by the fact that many elderly people have preexisting incontinence or dementia. *E. coli* is the number one cause of urinary tract infections, with *Staphylococcus saprophyticus* being second. Rarely, they may be due to viral or fungal infections. Other bacterial causes include: *Klebsiella*, *Proteus*, *Pseudomonas*, and *Enterobacter*. These are uncommon and typically related to abnormalities of the urinary system or urinary catheterization.

Urinary tract infections due to *Staphylococcus aureus* typically occurs secondary to blood born infections. In young sexually active women, sexual activity is the number one cause of bladder infections, with the risk of infection related to the frequency of sex. The term "honeymoon cystitis" has been applied to this phenomenon of frequent UTIs during early marriage. In post-menopausal women, sexual activity does not affect the risk of developing a UTI.

Spermicide use, independent of sexual frequency, increases the risk of UTIs. Women are more prone to UTIs than men because, in females, the urethra is much shorter and closer to the anus. As a woman's estrogen levels decrease with menopause, her risk of urinary tract infections increases due to the loss of protective vaginal flora. Urinary catheterization increases the risk for urinary tract infections. The risk of bacteriuria (bacteria in the urine) is between three to six percent per day and prophylactic antibiotics are not effective in decreasing symptomatic infections. The risk of an associated infection can be decreased by catheterizing only when necessary, using aseptic technique for insertion, and maintaining unobstructed closed drainage of the catheter. A predisposition for bladder infections may run in families.

Other risk factors include diabetes, being uncircumcised, and having a large prostate. Complicating factors are rather vague and include predisposing anatomic, functional, or metabolic abnormalities. Complicated UTI is more difficult to treat and usually requires more aggressive evaluation, treatment and follow-up.

In children, UTIs are associated with <u>constipation </u>and <u>vesicoureteral reflux</u> (an abnormal movement of urine from the bladder into ureters or kidneys. Persons with <u>spinal cord injury</u> are at increased risk for urinary tract infection in part because of chronic use of catheter, and in part because of <u>voiding</u> dysfunction. It is the most common cause of infection in this population, as well as the most common cause of hospitalization.

Nutritional factors: Home treatment of urinary tract infections often involves consuming and/or avoiding specific foods.

Hydration: Proper hydration helps the body flush out the bacteria. People with UTIs may notice they have to urinate much more often than normal. Drinking large quantities of water, unsweetened teas and similar drinks may help. Proper hydration encourages quicker healing. It also dilutes the urine, reducing discomfort while urinating. Additionally, use of cranberry juice or cranberry supplement appears to be ineffective in prevention and treatment in this population.

Antioxidants : Antioxidant foods, including tomatoes, cherries, blueberries and cranberries, etc., may encourage the body to heal more quickly. Cranberry juice is a traditional remedy for UTIs, and contains substances that prevent bacteria from living in bladder tissue. Regular consumption of <u>unsweetened cranberry juice</u> may even prevent UTIs from occurring. Herbal teas may help the body recover from a UTI more quickly. Low-caffeine green teas have antioxidant effects and may boost the immune system. Uva ursi, or bilberry, is a relative of the cranberry, and has similar effects. Taking both bilberry and cranberry together may help clear up a urinary tract infection more quick.

Vegetables, Vegetables of any kind will not only help relieve symptoms but also aid in the body recovering from a UTI more quickly.

Foods to Avoid: Some substances may aggravate UTI symptoms. Sweetened drinks, Caffeine, alcohol, and strong citrus drinks may irritate the bladder and urinary tract, and make urination more painful. Sweetened beverages may encourage bacterial growth and increase irritation so avoid refined carbohydrates. Also avoid red meat while suffering from a UTI.

URTICARIA: Urticaria (from the Latin urtica, nettle, and urere, to burn) commonly referred to as **hives**, is a kind of skin rash notable for pale red, raised, itchy bumps. They appear anywhere on the surface of the skin usually in response to an allergen or stress.

Signs and Symptoms: Appearance: wheals are raised areas surrounded by a red base. They can appear anywhere on the surface of the skin. Wheals may be pinpoint in size, or several inches in diameter. Angioedema is a related condition (also from allergic and non-allergic causes), though fluid leakage is from much deeper blood vessels. Individual hives that are painful, last more than 24 hours, or leave a bruise as they heal are more likely to be a more serious condition called urticarial vasculitis.

Cause: Whether the trigger is allergic or non-allergic, there is a complex release of inflammatory mediators, including histamine from cutaneous mast cells, resulting in fluid leakage from superficial blood vessels. Although hives are frequently caused by allergic reactions there are many non-allergic causes. Most cases of hives lasting less than six weeks (acute urticaria) are the result of an allergic trigger.

Chronic urticaria (hives lasting longer than six weeks) is rarely due to an allergy. The majority of patients with chronic hives have an unknown (idiopathic) cause. Perhaps as many as 30–40% of patients with chronic idiopathic urticaria will, in fact, have an autoimmune cause. Acute viral infection is another common cause of acute urticaria (viral exanthem). Less common causes of hives include friction, pressure, temperature extremes, exercise, and sunlight. Hives caused by stroking the skin (often linear in appearance) are due to a benign condition called dermographism.

Acute urticaria usually shows up a few minutes after contact with the allergen, and can last a few hours to several weeks. Food allergic reactions often fit in this category. Chronic urticaria refers to hives that persists for 6 weeks or more. There are no visual differences between acute and chronic urticaria. . Medicinal causes: The anti-diabetic sulphonylurea glimepiride (trade name Amaryl), in particular, has been documented to induce allergic reactions manifesting as urticaria. Other cases include dextroamphetamine, aspirin, ibuprofen, penicillin, clotrimazole, sulfonamides and anticonvulsants.

Nutritive factors: The most common food allergens are the proteins in cow's milk, eggs, peanuts, wheat, fish, shellfish and tree nuts. •Read food labels carefully and ask about ingredients, especially at restaurants or when eating food prepared by another person.

VARICOSE VEINS: Varicose veins are veins that have become enlarged and tortuous. The term commonly refers to the veins on the leg, although varicose veins can occur elsewhere. Veins have leaflet valves to prevent blood from flowing backwards (retrograde flow or reflux). Leg muscles pump the veins to return blood to the heart (the calf muscle pump mechanism), against the effects of gravity. When veins become varicose, the leaflets of the valves no longer meet properly, and the valves do not work (valvular incompetence). This allows blood to flow backwards and they enlarge even more. Varicose veins are most common in the superficial veins of the legs, which are subject to high pressure when standing. Besides being a cosmetic problem, varicose veins can be painful, especially when standing. Severe long-standing varicose veins can lead to leg swelling, venous eczema, skin thickening (lipodermatosclerosis) and ulceration. Life-threatening complications are uncommon.

Non-surgical treatments include sclerotherapy, elastic stockings, elevating the legs, and exercise. The traditional surgical treatment has been vein stripping to remove the affected veins. Newer, less invasive treatments which seal the main leaking vein are available. Alternative techniques, such as ultrasound-guided foam sclerotherapy, radiofrequency ablation and endovenous laser treatment, are available as well.

Because most of the blood in the legs is returned by the deep veins, the superficial veins, which return only about 10 per cent of the total blood of the legs, can usually be removed or ablated without serious harm. Secondary varicose veins are those developing as collateral pathways, typically after stenosis or occlusion of the deep veins, a common sequel of extensive deep venous thrombosis (DVT). Treatment options are usually support stockings, occasionally sclerotherapy, and rarely limited surgery.

Varicose veins are distinguished from reticular veins (blue veins) and telangiectasias (spider veins), which also involve valvular insufficiency, by the size and location of the veins. Many patients who suffer with varicose veins seek out the assistance of physicians who specialize in vein care or pheripheral vascular disease. These physicians are called Vascular Surgeons, phlebologists or interventional radiologists.

Signs and Symptoms

> ➢ Aching, heavy legs (often worse at night and after exercise).

> ➤ Appearance of spider veins (telangiectasia) in the affected leg.
> ➤ Ankle swelling, especially in evening.
> ➤ A brownish-blue shiny skin discoloration near the affected veins.
> ➤ Redness, dryness, and itchiness of areas of skin, termed stasis dermatitis or venous eczema, because of waste products building up in the leg.
> ➤ Cramps may develop especially when making a sudden move as standing up.
> ➤ Minor injuries to the area may bleed more than normal and/or take a long time to heal.
> ➤ In some people the skin above the ankle may shrink (lipodermatosclerosis) because the fat underneath the skin becomes hard.
> ➤ Restless legs syndrome appears to be a common overlapping clinical syndrome in patients with varicose veins and other chronic venous insufficiency.
> ➤ Whitened, irregular scar-like patches at the ankles is known as atrophie blanche.

Investigations: Traditionally, varicose veins were only investigated using imaging techniques if there was a clinical suspicion of deep venous insufficiency, if they were recurrent, or if they involved the sapheno-popliteal junction. This practice is not now widely accepted. All patients with varicose veins should now be investigated using Duplex doppler ultrasound scanning. The results from a randomized controlled trial (RCT) on the follow up of patients with and without routine Duplex scan has shown a significant difference in recurrence rate and reoperation rate at 2 years of follow up.

Complications: Most varicose veins are relatively benign, but severe varicosities can lead to major complications, due to the poor circulation through the affected limb.

- ✓ Pain, heaviness, inability to walk or stand for long hours, thus hindering work
- ✓ Skin conditions: e.g., Stasis Dermatitis which could predispose skin loss
- ✓ Skin ulcers especially near the ankle, usually referred to as venous ulcers.
- ✓ Development of carcinoma or sarcoma in longstanding venous ulcers.
- ✓ Severe bleeding from minor trauma, of particular concern in the elderly.
- ✓ Blood clotting within affected veins is termed superficial thrombophlebitis. These are frequently isolated to the superficial veins, but can extend into deep veins becoming a more serious problem.
- ✓ Acute fat necrosis can occur, especially at the ankle of overweight patients with varicose veins. Females are more frequently affected than males.
- ✓ The afflicted person suffers tenderness in that region

Causes: Varicose veins are more common in women than in men, and are linked with heredity. Other related factors are pregnancy, obesity, menopause, aging, prolonged standing, leg injury, abdominal straining, and crossing legs at the knees or ankles. Less commonly, but not exceptionally, varicose veins can be due to other causes, as post phlebitic obstruction and/or incontinence, venous and arteriovenous malformations.

Foods that can Prevent and/or Cure Varicose Veins: All of these factors can be improved through food making it possible to prevent and treat varicose veins.

Fiber: Foods that are high in fiber help maintain many healthy body systems but are particularly important for improving varicose veins. By regulating the colon and digestion, fiber prevents the build-up of toxins in the blood and keeps it flowing regularly. This then, keeps the blood pumping back to the heart instead of pooling near the skin. Steamed spinach is a great source of fiber as are beans, whole grains and carrots. Red beets and beet juice are also useful for avoiding blood toxemia.

Dissolving Calcium Deposits: Varicose veins are also attributed to inorganic calcium accumulating in the veins. This build up blocks the blood's upward movement like a dam, forcing the veins to bulge outwards near the skins surface. Raw garlic is known to dissolve deposits of both inorganic calcium and cholesterol, allowing the blood to flow freely. Parsley, on the other hand, not only dissolves calcium in the veins, it improves oxygen metabolism and helps maintain the elasticity of blood vessels. This makes parsley one of the best food choices for someone with varicose veins.

Vitamin C and Flavonoids: Free radicals often cause damage to veins and weaken them. Therefore, foods that are high in flavonoids which reduce free radicals can be used to treat and prevent varicose veins. Dark greens such as spinach, dark fruits such as cherries and blueberries, yams, onions, grapes and dark chocolate are all good sources of these antioxidants. In addition, acerola cherries provide the full vitamin C complex. This makes it a double dose of varicose fighting power because vitamin C strengthens the vein walls. To get vitamin C, try eating citrus or bell peppers. And all of these fruits and vegetables provide more nutrients if juiced and eaten raw.

Tannins/Rutins: Spinach not only provides flavonoids, it also contains tannins. Tannins tighten and strengthen the tissue of the veins in the way that they are also used to "tan" leather. Another potent source of tannins is horse chestnut, an herb that doctors in Europe now prescribe for varicose veins. Dark greens also contain some tannin, buckwheat greens having the highest level.

Foods to Avoid: When treating varicose veins through diet, avoiding certain foods is necessary to promote the health of the veins. Refined sugar and refined flour are both detrimental to the cardiovascular system, e.g., Eating popular store items such as cookies, doughnuts, candy and many boxed cereals will negate the effects of the beneficial foods and trigger any or all of the metabolic medical diseases controlled by insulin.

APPENDIX I: ANTIOXIDANT FOODS

FOODS CONTAINING ANTI-OXIDANTS ARE ALSO GOOD ANTI-AGING NUTRIENTS

Vitamin C:
  Citrus fruits
  Berries
  Tomatoes
  Peppers
  Cabbage
  Broccoli
  Brussels Sprouts
  Cauliflower
  Cantaloupe
Vitamin E:
  Vegetable oils (is rich in vitamin E)
  Wheat and other cereal grains
  Green leafy vegetables
  Egg yolk
  Milk fat
  Butter, real
  Meat
  Nuts
  Organ Meats
  Seafood
  Avocados
Vitamin A:
  Liver
  Egg yolks
  Whole milk
  Carrots
  Sweet potato
  Kale Turnip greens
  Mustard greens
  Pink Grapefruit
  Broccoli
  Cantaloupe
  Apricots
  Beet greens

Collard greens:
Papaya
Red Peppers
Cheddar cheese

Zinc:
Lean meat
Seafood
Eggs
Green leafy vegetables
Soybeans
Peanuts
Whole Bran
Whole cereals
Cheese

Lutein and Zeaxanthin:
Kale
Collard greens
Spinach
Celery
Broccoli
Lettuce
Green peas
Pumpkin
Brussels sprouts
Summer squash
Corn
Green beans
Green peppers
Cucumbers
Green olives

Note: It is often quoted, "**we are what we eat**", There is no better way to get healthy and stay healthy than to include anti-inflammatory and anti-oxidant food nutrients in your daily diet.

APPENDIX II: DETOXIFICATION

Detoxification is about resting, cleaning and nourishing the body from the inside out. By removing and eliminating toxins from the blood, then feeding our body with healthy nutrients, detoxifying can help protect us from disease, even many cancers and renew your ability to maintain optimum health. It does this mainly by removing impurities from the blood via the liver, where toxins are detoxified. The body can then eliminate these "detoxified - toxins" through the kidneys, intestines/colon, lungs, lymph and skin. However, when any of these systems are compromised, impurities (toxins) aren't properly detoxified and every cell in the body is adversely affected. Detoxification enhances the body's own natural healing systems.

Detoxification is one of the many functions of the liver. The liver combines toxic substances, such as drugs, alcohol, metabolic waste and environmental toxins with substances that are less toxic to produce a neutralized substance. This neutralized substance is then excreted through the skin, kidneys, lungs and/or bowel. Certain nutritional drinks and/or foods can help cleanse the liver and can repair and heal damaged tissues, cells and cell receptors and thus these nutrients are needed to maintain good health.

The best way to get healthy is to work from the inside out starting with the cleansing (detoxification) of the liver. <u>Putting the proper nutrients into your body is always important, but first you want to flush out the toxins or poisons</u>. The toxins that build up in the body usually are notice first in your skin, causing it to look rough and dull and your body, in general, to look puffy. <u>Toxic chemicals are poisonous</u>. Toxic chemicals cause inflammation and it is the chronic build up of inflammatory injury that causes many of our modern day medical diseases.

If your system is clean and free of toxic, poisonous chemicals that inflame and therefore cause damage to cells: then and only then can the good nutrients you put into your body finally get to where they belong. Then you can be a more energetic, beautiful and healthy.

A detox program can help the body's natural cleaning process by:

1) Resting the organs through fasting:

2) Stimulating the liver to detoxify and eliminate toxins from the body:

3) Promoting elimination of these toxins through the intestines, kidneys and skin:

4) Improving circulation of the blood: and

5) Refueling the body with healthy nutrients.

There are many everyday natural foods that are great for helping the liver detoxify and cleanse the body. Many are listed below.

1. Seaweed. "Sea Crackers". Seaweed is a fabulous detox food because it contains a variety of vital minerals and nutrients from the sea. The nutrients contained in sea vegetation bind with and remove harmful toxins from the body. "Brown Algae" is a good example of a sea weed that has purifying properties.

2. Garlic. Garlic is known as a blood purifier. It has powerful detox properties. Garlic has several antioxidants that are very effective in cleansing the blood. Garlic is also known as a natural cholesterol lowering supplement.

3. Apple Cider Vinegar. Long used for its purifying properties, apple cider vinegar is a natural way to purify your body. The benefits of

apple cider vinegar include: Supports a healthy immune system: Helps control weight: Promotes digestion: Helps soothe dry throats. Helps remove toxins that cause sludge and damage: and Balance the acid base system (ph). One method is to ingest a Tbsp of apple cider vinegar in the morning as a cleansing to your digestive system. Apple Cider Vinegar is unfiltered, unheated, unpasteurized and 5% acidity.

4. Spirulina. The sprulina contains many nutrients and can boost nutrition during a detox phase. Dried spirulina contains about 60% (51–71%) protein. It is a complete protein containing all essential amino acids. It is superior to typical plant protein, such as that from legumes.

5. Apples. I am separating apples as a special purifying food. Apples contain high amounts of pectin and fiber. This is a perfect de-tox combo to digest. Always try to choose organic apples. And always eat the skin-that's where most the vitamins are hiding!

6. High Fiber, Raw Fruits and Veggies. Raw fruits and veggies are by far the BEST purifying foods out there. Fiber is incredibly cleansing to you digestive system. Produce that is raw and high in fiber will certainly assist your body in its natural detoxification processes. Examples of fruits and veggies that are high in fiber and nutrients include: spinach, apples, oranges, citrus, carrots, kale, papaya, bananas, pineapple, figs, romaine, watercress, parsley, arugula, blackberries, blueberries and strawberries...just to name a few.

7. Cayenne and Ginger. Add a sprinkle of cayenne to your juice or smoothie and you will get an instant warming sensation. The spicy kick will jump start your metabolism. Stimulating foods and ingredients like ginger, cayenne and pepper are all great for detox and purification.

8. Lemon Juice. Lemon juice is similar to apple cider vinegar for purification. The acidity helps to purify and cleanse the colon,

while the acid helps to break up any food, toxins or nutrients hanging out in your digestive system. Adding a squeeze of lemon to your tea in the morning, or even to a warm glass of water first thing in the morning is a good way to use lemon as a detox aid. And if you are really brave-try a lemon-apple-cayenne-ginger juice first thing in the morning. Super stimulating (and yummy).

9. Grapefruit. Another favorite detox food of many is grapefruit. It's packed with fiber-especially if the white stuff just beneath the rind is also consumed. It's deliciously sweet and tangy. And it has a nice dose of nutrients, especially vitamin C.

10. Probiotics and Yogurt. Whenever you are taking extra steps to detox your body of toxins and sweep away some of that bad bacteria in your colon, you have to remember that the more good bacteria you have the better off you are. I highly recommend find yummy brand of soy yogurt that you like and can get in the habit of eating daily. And if you don't mind spending a few extra bucks, Bio-K Plus is an amazing brand with dairy-free soy yogurt shots. It is the most powerful vegan yogurt shot on the market. I buy mine at Whole Foods. You can also take supplements, but I personally hate popping pills unless it's completely necessary.

11. Warm Lemon Water: Lemons are a super-food - rich in potassium, vitamin C and citric acid. Warm water and lemon, is known as a lemon tonic. Drinking warm lemon water cleanses the liver and also has a positive effect on the bile and the digestive system.

12. Broccoli and Cabbage Juice: Broccoli and cabbage are cruciferous vegetables that can be juiced into a liver cleansing drink. They enhance liver detoxification by their active ingredient, indoles. Indoles are phytonutrients that help detoxify the body. Cruciferous vegetables provide a rich source of indoles. These include Brussels sprouts, broccoli, bok choy, cabbage and turnips.

Studies show that consuming a high dietary intake of cruciferous vegetables and berries will also decrease cancer risks. Indoles are shown to exert anti-carcinogen activity. Indole-3-carbinol inhibits prostate cancer cells and can help prevent prostate cancer it can also treat prostate cancer. Other studies have found similar results with breast cancer and colon cancer also. You should consult your health-care provider before increasing your cruciferous vegetable intake if you have a thyroid disorder. Cruciferous vegetables are known as goitrogens, which are foods that can suppress thyroid function so one should always be careful and not over do it in one specific element or ingredient of nutritional food. Balance is still the key to good health. Eating a diet rich in fruits, vegetables and whole grains will not only help to reduce your risk of cancer they will help prevent and treat other diseases.

13. Dandelion Tea: Dandelion contains nutrients, such as calcium, magnesium, iron, selenium, zinc, phosphorous and vitamins B and C. The dandelion root contains bitter crystalline compounds called "Taraxacin". In addition, the root contains compounds called "inulin and levulin". Together, these compounds are responsible for the healing properties of the herb. Dandelions can be boiled into a therapeutic tea that cleanses the liver.

14. Fruit Smoothies: certain fresh fruits help to stimulate energy flow through the liver, enhancing its function. Blackberries, strawberries, blueberries and raspberries are considered liver fruits. These healthy and potent berries make a delicious liver cleansing fruit smoothie, especially when combined with a banana and almond milk.

15. Bananas: Another example of a nutritious medicinal food is the banana. Bananas are one of the most popular foods and for good reason. Bananas are filled with Potassium: giving your body the ability to handle stress, maintain a healthy blood pressure and provide sustained energy - the healthy way without any harmful

side effects. Bananas keep the heart and the nervous system in shape not to mention the advantages of its nutrients that keep muscles strong. Bananas also help keep the bones strong and the kidneys and blood functioning better by regulating and maintaining the right acid-base balance. Basically, bananas are a good choice as a snack or with a meal. Whether you run walk or ride a bike, the Banana is very important to the body.   Banana Smoothie: Need a quick energy boost while on the go, try a tasty Banana smoothie. Protect your nervous system from the stress of the day, strengthen your muscles and reduce your blood pressure and cholesterol by drinking this delicious snack. The banana is naturally sweet helping you to avoid the other sweet things that may not be so good for you.

16. Nutmeg can clean both your liver and kidneys and remove many toxins.

17. Celery juice is a good because it has "natural" sodium, i.e. the same content of sodium as human blood (0.09%). If the saline level in your body is not kept within a healthy range you can become dehydrated causing hypernatremia or over-hydrated causing hyponatremia. The salt in celery helps our bodies utilize the nutrients that are put into it. Celery also deletes carbon dioxide from the body and therefore celery can regulate the acid build up in the body. Celery has a great deal of fiber that helps control the absorption of dietary sugars and cholesterol. Celery also helps the body to regulate temperature. Arteries can become hardened when there is too much calcium and bad cholesterol in the body and celery can reduce the calcium naturally because it contains the right amount of sodium. Celery is also good for the colon (digestive system) because it is also a colon cleanser. The nutrients in celery can also stimulate the elimination of urine from the body, and therefore celery acts as a diuretic. Celery is also a calming agent that is good for treating anxiety or other nervous disorders. Celery has been used for its medicinal powers for centuries. It is best to

juice celery. However, celery is good cooked in soups and stews or eaten raw in salads. Celery is a food that basically brings the body back to normal. When the body is in balance and we maintain it properly, it works better.

Note: Raw foods work the best for detoxifying. Raw fresh pressed juices (like celery, lemon, grapefruit, oranges, etc.) and smoothies (like a blueberry-spirulina smoothie) are just a few of the ways to detoxify. Also, choose raw nuts and seeds over roasted and live raw salads instead of cooked veggies. Going raw for a few days will boost the live enzymes in your system, give you a lot of cleansing natural fiber and give you energy. Eating raw foods 100%

Biography - Carla Denise Oldenberg Sharbono, M.D.

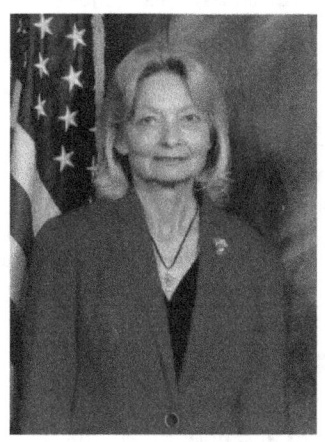

Denise is a retired medical doctor who has renewed her interest in writing. She specializes in subjects related to medicine, nutrition, safe and effective means of weight loss. After more than 20 years as a practicing family physician, she has retired to the Mountain Home area of Arkansas to begin a "physician guided weight loss program" that focuses on good nutrition and healthy life style changes that will be beneficial in not only correcting health problems but will also help individuals achieve their ideal weight and a healthier life style and therefore prevent many of today's age-related metabolic medical diseases.

Born in Billings, Montana, Denise graduated in 1965 from Huntley Project High School in Worden, Montana. She then joined the U.S. Marine Corps and served her country from 1965 – 1968. After finishing her military obligation she used the GI Bill to obtain a college education. She received her BS degree in Health and Physical Education with a minor in Chemistry and Biology and began teaching high school science in 1971. She taught school for 7 years in Louisiana. However, when one of her students was accepted into medical school, she realized she could also become a medical doctor. She enjoyed teaching but wanted to help people, one-on-one, with the knowledge she had gained. As a classroom teacher with class sizes of 24 to 30 students: she felt she was more of a disciplinarian than a teacher.

Denise received her M.D. degree in 1986 from Louisiana State University Medical Center in Shreveport, La. In 1988 she received her Arkansas medical license and then moved to Arkansas where she began her medical practice in rural Arkansas, between Dover and Witt Springs. She also worked as an Emergency Room Physician in various small hospitals throughout northern Arkansas from 1995 to 2003. In 1998 she moved her medical practice to the Salem, Horseshoe Bend and the Cherokee Village area of Arkansas where she not only kept her clinic opened but continued to work in the Salem and Cherokee Village Hospitals as one of their ER physicians. She also delivered babies at the Salem hospital from 1998 until 2002. This was during the (time) when rural hospitals could obtain malpractice insurance for family physicians doing obstetrics as well as a time that family physicians could afford malpractice in obstetrics.

Her mission still remains "to serve others" by teaching or instructing them on how they can become a healthier individual by using natural (food) nutrients. She believes good nutrition and a healthy weight are at the core of achieving this goal for all individuals. By achieving a healthy weight and eating healthy (food) nutrients, (avoiding sugar, nonnutritive artificial sweeteners and hydrogenated oils or trans-fats, i.e., margarine and shortening and processed foods made with these "trans-fats"), she believes individuals can prevent, treat and even cure many of their own health problems. For example, stress management and poor nutritional eating are known to be risk factors that contribute to anxiety, arthritis, diabetes, hypertension, heart disease due to high cholesterol/high triglyceride eye disease, depression, acid reflux (GERD), neurological diseases and chronic pain issues, etc. Knowledge about good nutrition and safe and effective weight loss as well as how to handle stress will be the center of focus at each encounter.

Denise is the proud and happy mother of 2 adult children and a grandmother. Also, Denise is a proud Marine and a member of Twin Lakes Marine and the Marine Corps League. As a veteran of the Vietnam era she continues to help veterans, through diet, counseling and medication, who deal with post traumatic issues and depression, overcome some of the issues that hinder them from achieving a better quality of life.

www.ingramcontent.com/pod-product-compliance
Lightning Source LLC
Chambersburg PA
CBHW060451290526
45791CB00001B/75